'BEST OF FIVE' CLINICAL SCENARIOS FOR THE MRCP

COMING SOON

"BEST OF FIVE" CLINICAL SCENARIOS FOR THE MRCP PART 1 – VOLUME 2

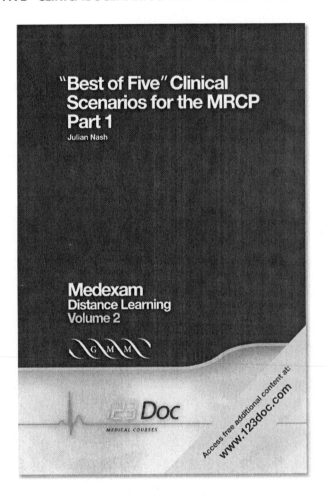

Edited by Julian Nash

Volume 2 covers the remaining Part 1 topics...

- Biochemistry
- Cell and Molecular Medicine
- Clinical Pharmacology
- Endocrine and Metabolic Medicine
- Genetics
- Immunology
- Rheumatology
- Statistics and Epidemiology

'BEST OF FIVE'
CLINICAL SCENARIOS FOR THE MRCP

by
Punit Ramrakha

MA (Cambridge), BMBCh (Oxon), MRCP (UK), PhD (London)
*Consultant Cardiologist, Stoke Mandeville Hospital, Aylesbury
and Hammersmith Hospital, London*

Iqbal Malik

MBBChir (Cambridge), MA (Cambridge), MRCP (UK)
*Consultant Cardiologist, St Mary's Hospital
London*

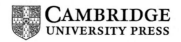
CAMBRIDGE
UNIVERSITY PRESS

CAMBRIDGE UNIVERSITY PRESS

Cambridge, New York, Melbourne, Madrid, Cape Town, Singapore, São Paulo

Cambridge University Press
The Edinburgh Building, Cambridge CB2 2RU, UK

Published in the United States of America by Cambridge University Press, New York

www.cambridge.org
Information on this title: www.cambridge.org/9780521676786

First published 2004
Reprinted by Cambridge University Press 2005

Printed in the United Kingdom at the University Press, Cambridge

A catalogue record for this publication is available from the British Library

Typeset by Mizpah Publishing Services, Chennai, India

ISBN-13 978-0-521-67678-6 paperback
ISBN-10 0-521-67678-9 paperback

Contents

Preface

The Membership of the Royal College of Physicians (MRCP) is a major milestone for physicians in training. The examination has evolved, and the Royal College of Physicians has modified the exam format to be more relevant to the clinical care of patients while still testing the basic knowledge of Medicine.

The recent change in examination format has made the revision books and materials published over the years largely obsolete. This new book is based on the new form of MCQ – 'Best Of Five' Clinical Scenarios, matching the style and standards set by the College.

The material is divided by specialty, and highlights topics in each specialty with examples of questions on the topic. While space does not permit us to cover the entire syllabus in one volume, this book contains eight chapters covering eight specialties and a total of 225 questions. This is the first in a series of books designed to complement each other and provide students with a comprehensive revision guide for the examination.

A revolutionary 'Distance learning solution'

The exam requires a very broad knowledge of medicine which one can only acquire by reading additional reference material and in medical practice. But the MCQs question format set a difficult task in revision: study material in textbooks and patients on the wards do not come in the multiple choice format, and the skills of being a good doctor do not directly translate to answering the MCQs correctly. The examination is competitive, has a high failure rate, and unfortunately for many, even Part 1 can be a disheartening obstacle while in an SHO job, with nights on-call and long, restless hours on the ward.

For these reasons, 123Doc Medical Courses has developed a revolutionary new concept of revision aids for the candidates of the MRCP Part 1, a 'distance learning' solution combining the traditional use of a book with the flexibility and interactivity of the internet. The Medexam series has been conceived so that doctors who purchase this book can experience all of the benefits of 123Doc's celebrated courses as well as of a book, and access additional interactive services and content online, making the best use of their time.

You will find on the back cover of this book, a scratch card that will provide you with a 'passkey' to access this book from 123Doc's website. Once logged on to www.123doc.com, your personal 'passkey' will allow you to benefit from the interactivity of the 123doc online study.

Access additional resources in a click:

Traditional books of MCQs often raise further questions in the reader: what are the other causes of this symptom, what is this disease all about, etc. The reader then has to find a textbook of medicine and search through the index to find the information, perhaps requiring several books to find all the answers.

On www.123doc.com, all the questions of this textbook have been linked to 123doc's online medical resource. Besides the teaching notes, additional material, from simple lists to relevant sections from the online textbooks, can be accessed in a 'click' to get a broader view of a topic. Each of these layers of content brings different depths of information and serves a different purpose, catering for the fact that each student has different previous knowledge than his or her fellows.

Furthermore, www.123doc.com's user-friendly facilities allow you to search by keyword so that you can easily retrieve questions by topic.

Forgetting to carry your revision book is no longer an obstacle and you will be able to continue revisions from any computer at any time (on call, at work, at home, when visiting boring relatives, etc).

A virtual community:

123Doc e-books give you access to a virtual community of people, which should bring you the same benefits as that of a classroom community:

You will be able to email our online tutors and ask questions to clear up your doubts as well as to receive regular exam-related newsletters to keep you updated with the College's syllabus and question format.

Most importantly, you will be able to test yourself by taking timed mock exams, and receive a score as well as a rating against other students who took a mock exam under similar conditions. These mock exams are essential to your preparation, as you will learn how to pace yourself and be efficient during the exam. The automatic scoring and rating system allows you to assess whether you are ready to sit the exam or whether you should keep studying.

The key to success is to plan your time carefully, not trying to learn all of Medicine before the examination, but studying in a way that prepares you for that specific examination. As with all exams based on MCQs, practice is the key – to acquire knowledge, identify gaps and learn the technique to answering the questions to maximise your score. This book and the related online services through www.123doc.com will allow you to do that.

Good luck!

Sabine Guerry
Co-founder and CEO
123Doc Medical Courses
October 2003

Contributors

Chapter 1: Cardiology
Dr Iqbal Malik
MBBChir (Cambridge), MA (Cambridge), MRCP (UK)
Consultant Cardiologist
St Mary's Hospital
London

Chapter 2: Dermatology
Dr Vandana S. Ramrakha-Jones
MA (Hons), BMBCh (Oxon), MRCP (UK)
Specialist Registrar in Dermatology
Glasgow Royal Infirmary

Chapter 3: Gastroenterology
Geoff Smith
BSc MRCP (UK)
Specialist Registrar in Gastroenterology
University College Hospitals
Honorary Research Fellow
St Bart's and the London School of Medicine
London

Chapter 4: Haematology
Dr Joanna Howard
MA (Cambridge), MBBChir (Cambridge), MRCP (UK), MRCPath
Consultant Haematologist
Central Middlesex Hospital
London

Chapter 5: Infectious Diseases
Dr David Wareham
MB BS MSc MRCP(UK), DipRCPath DTM&H DGM
Clinical Training Fellow and Honorary SpR in Medical Microbiology
Queen Mary's School of Medicine and Dentisty and Barts &
The London NHS Trust
London

Chapter 6: Nephrology
Dr Ashik Sainu K.M.
Registrar in Nephrology
General Medical Centre Hospital
Abu Dhabi, UAE

Chapter 7: Neurology
Dr Parashkev Nachev
MA (Cambridge), BM BCh (Oxon), MRCP(UK)
Clinical Research Fellow, Department of Neuroscience
Imperial College
London

Chapter 8: Respiratory Medicine
Dr Harsha Kariyawasam
BSc(hons), MBBS MRCP(UK)
Specialist Registrar in Respiratory Medicine
Royal Brompton Hospital
London

Contributors

Editors Profile

Dr Punit Ramrakha
MA (Cambridge), BMBCh (Oxon), MRCP (UK), PhD (London)
Consultant Cardiologist, Stoke Mandeville Hospital, Aylesbury
and Hammersmith Hospital, London

Punit graduated from Cambridge (MA, 1st Class Hons.) and Oxford University (BMBCh) with many university prizes. He has trained in General Medicine at Hammersmith Hospital, Royal Brompton Hospital, St Thomas's Hospital and National Hospital Queen Square in London, before undertaking his cardiology training as a Registrar at the Hammersmith Hospital, Charing Cross Hospital and St Mary's Hospital, London. He has a good foundation in Molecular Medicine and the Basic Sciences, and spent 4 years doing a PhD into endothelial adhesion molecules; he received University and International Awards for this work. He was appointed as Consultant Cardiologist in 2002.

Punit has extensive experience in writing and teaching: he is Editor of the Oxford Handbook of Clinical Medicine 3rd Edition (OUP, 1993), the Oxford Handbook of Acute Medicine (OUP, 1997), and QBase Medicine 1 (GMM, 1998). He has been teaching on courses for the MRCP and MRCPCH in London since 1994 and co-founded 123Doc Medical Courses in 2000.

Dr Iqbal Malik
MBBChir (Cambridge), MA (Cambridge), MRCP (UK)
Consultant Cardiologist, St Mary's Hospital, London

Iqbal trained at Peterhouse, Cambridge University, where he was a Scholar and gained a 1st class honours degree. He then completed his undergraduate education at Guy's Hospital, London, winning several prizes along the way. His postgraduate education was on the Royal London Senior House Officer Rotation, before he became a Registrar in Cardiology at the Hammersmith Hospital. Having worked at several West London Hospitals, he was appointed as a Consultant Interventional Cardiologist at St Mary's Hospital, London, in 2003. He completed his PhD thesis in 2003 looking at inflammatory markers in coronary heart disease. He has published several papers on the role of inflammation.

Iqbal has been involved in undergraduate and postgraduate education since 1995, teaching medical students, MRCP candidates and specialist trainees. In addition, he is involved in innovative training programs for general practitioners and non-medical specialists.

Cardiology

Abnormalities of the ECG

Q 1. A 24-year-old professional footballer is referred for a medical prior to being signed-up for a team. Which of the following features of his resting ECG would suggest cardiac disease?

   A. T-wave inversion in V1–V5
   B. Wenckebach phenomenon
   C. Junctional rhythm at rest of 45 beats per minute
   D. Voltage criteria for left ventricular hypertrophy (LVH)
   E. Dominant R wave in lead V1

Q 2. On a 12-lead ECG, ST elevation in the chest leads may be seen with all of the following except:

   A. Hyperkalaemia
   B. Syndrome X
   C. Ventricular aneurysm
   D. Hypertrophic cardiomyopathy (HCM)
   E. Subarachnoid haemorrhage

A 1.   A

The resting ECG in an athlete reflects the high vagal tone, so that bradycardia, Wenckebach phenomenon, junctional rhythm and first-degree heart block may occur. In addition, RBBB can be a normal finding in a young adult, leading to a dominant R wave in lead V1. However, widespread T-wave inversion is not normal, and may reflect abnormal LVH or ischaemia.

A 2.   B

ST elevation is a marker for coronary occlusion, but may also occur with pericarditis, ventricular aneurysm, Printzmetal angina (spasm), and rarely with hyperkalaemia and subarachnoid haemorrhage. High take off in leads with deep S waves can cause ST elevation in hypertrophic cardiomyopathy (HCM). Syndrome X is associated with ST depression and angiographically normal coronary arteries.

Causes of dominant 'R' in V1
- RBBB
- Right ventricular hypertrophy
- Dextrocardia
- True posterior infarction
- Wolf-Parkinson-White Syndrome Type A (left sided pathway)
- Duchene muscular dystrophy

JVP, Pulse, and Heart Sounds

Q 3. A 39-year-old woman presents with breathlessness. On examination she is noted to have a wide split and fixed second heart sound. Which of the following is the most likely diagnosis?

    A. Fallot's tetralogy

    B. Constrictive pericarditis

    C. Aortic stenosis

    D. RBBB

    E. Secundum atrial septal defect

Q 4. Causes of a reversed split second heart sound include:

    A. Right bundle branch block (RBBB)

    B. Left bundle branch block (LBBB)

    C. Right atrial pacing

    D. Mild aortic stenosis

    E. Ventricular septal defect

A 3.　E

The second heart sound is made up of the closure of the aortic valve (A2), followed by the closure of the pulmonary valve (P2). P2 is delayed on inspiration as there is more blood flowing into the right heart, hence physiological splitting. P2 is delayed even on expiration if there is RBBB, getting wider still on inspiration, unless the RBBB is accompanied by a connection between the two atria, as in an atrial septal defect, hence wide fixed splitting.

A 4.　B

S2 is reversed split if at rest P2 occurs before A2. Then with inspiration, as P2 is delayed, the gap between the two components of S2 gets smaller. This may occur with delay in A2, as with severe aortic stenosis (not mild), left bundle branch block and right ventricular pacing.

Wide split second heart sound
- Fixed split – ASD
- Delayed P2
  - RBBB
  - Pulmonary stenosis
- Early A2
  - Severe mitral regurgitation
  - VSD

Myocardial Disease

Q 5. A 46-year-old man with a history of high alcohol intake presents with breathlessness and peripheral oedema. Which of the following feature would not be characteristic of alcoholic cardiomyopathy?

A. Dilated cardiomyopathy
B. Mitral regurgitation
C. Pericardial effusion
D. Increased risk of arrhythmias
E. Improvement with thiamine replacement

Q 6. The following are of aetiological significance in defining the cause of a cardiomyopathy:

A. T-wave flattening in the inferior ECG leads in a 60-year-old man
B. The presence of a soft pan-systolic murmur in the mitral area
C. AST of 50 IU/l with a bilirubin of 12 μmol/l in a 50-year-old lady
D. The presence of sinus tachycardia, with BP 140/80
E. The presence of diabetes mellitus in a tanned patient

A 5. **C**

Chronic alcohol abuse results in myocyte mitochondrial damage and a dilated cardiomyopathy. An elevated γ-GT or MCV would be suggestive of ethanol toxicity as a cause. This particular cardiomyopathy may be improved with thiamine. As with other dilated cardiomyopathies, mitral regurgitation and arrhythmias are common.

A 6. **E**

The commonest form of cardiomyopathy is dilated cardiomyopathy, with dilatation of the left ventricle, and reduction in the ejection fraction. No cause is often found, although rarely, it can be familial. A cause should be looked for in most cases. The commonest causes are ischaemic heart disease (Q-waves on the ECG, history of MI), and hypertension. Non-specific ECG changes and atrial fibrillation are common and do not point to a specific cause. Minor abnormalities of liver function result from liver congestion. More marked abnormalities and diabetes in a pigmented patient would suggest haemochromatosis. Mitral regurgitation and arrhythmias are common in dilated cardiomyopathy of any cause.

Haemochromatosis
- AR
- Chromosome 6-HFE gene in 80%
- Bronzing diabetes
- Hypogonadotrophic hypogonadism
- Iron overload with cirrhosis
- Dilated cardiomyopathy
- Joint problems
- Treat by regular phlebotomy
- 1 unit blood removes 250 mg iron

Evidence Based Cardiology

Q 7. **In congestive cardiac failure, which of the following drugs has not proven benefit in reducing overall mortality?**

  A. Angiotensin converting enzyme inhibitors
  B. Spironolactone
  C. Bisoprolol
  D. Hydralazine with nitrates
  E. Frusemide

Q 8. **In patients with ischaemic heart disease (IHD) all the following are true except:**

  A. A fall in blood pressure on exercise testing suggests severe coronary disease
  B. The only finding on examination may be a fourth heart sound during an acute attack
  C. Dyspnoea after an attack of angina is the hallmark of poor left ventricular (LV) function
  D. Angiotensin converting enzyme inhibitor (ACE-I) therapy reduces myocardial infarction rates
  E. A positive troponin-T without creatinine kinase (CK) rise diagnoses non-Q wave myocardial infarction

A 7. E

Diuretics do not prolong life in the long term. Trials in heart failure have shown that ACE-I are better than the combination of nitrates and hydralazine, which are better than placebo, in prolonging survival in heart failure. β-blockers (bisoprolol, metoprolol and carvedilol) and spironolactone have also shown a mortality advantage.

A 8. C

Ischaemic heart disease is often manifesting only with the symptoms of angina. Examination may find predisposing factors (e.g. hypertension), or complications (e.g. heart failure), but in the absence of these, a fourth heart sound during an attack of angina may be the only finding. Even before systolic LV dysfunction occurs, cardiac ischaemia produces diastolic dysfunction, causing impaired relaxation and a stiff ventricle, creating the conditions for an S4 with atrial systole. The myocardium can become 'stunned' with ischaemia, so causing temporary LV systolic impairment and dyspnoea despite good resting LV function. The use of ACE-I is associated with reduced future MI rates as shown in the HOPE trial. The definition of non-Q wave myocardial infarction has expanded to include those patients with unstable angina who have had a rise in troponin-T only. Their prognosis is as bad whether or not CK is also elevated.

Trials in heart failure
- ACE-I – SAVE, SOLVE, CONSENSUS
- β-blockers – CIBIS, CIBIS-II
- Spironolactone – Rales
- Hydralazine and nitrates – VHEFT-I
- Angiotensin receptor blockers – no mortality advantage but additive morbidity reduction on top of ACE-I – VAL-HFT

Congenital Valvular Disease

Q 9. A 32-year-old man is noted to have a systolic murmur at an insurance medical. Blood pressure is normal. An echocardiogram shows a bicuspid aortic valve. Which of the following are recognised associations?

A. Calcification of the valve in childhood
B. Triple vessel coronary disease in adulthood
C. Coarctation of the aorta
D. Marfan's syndrome
E. Left main stem anomalous origin in 2% of cases

Q 10. The following are true for mitral valve prolapse except:

A. It is associated with atrial septal defect
B. The murmur is louder and shorter on squatting
C. It is associated with a mutation in the gene for desmin
D. It has an increased risk of endocarditis
E. It is associated with long-QT syndrome

A 9. C

Bicuspid aortic valve occurs in 1–2% of the population. It may remain asymptomatic but can become stenotic or regurgitant with time. It is associated with a left dominant coronary circulation (i.e. the posterior descending artery arises from the left circumflex rather than the right coronary artery). 5% of cases demonstrate significant coarctation of the aorta. Calcification does not occur until adult life, and unlike calcific aortic stenosis of the old, coronary disease is very rare.

A 10. C

Mitral valve prolapse appears to be associated with most cardiac problems, including endocarditis, atrial septal defect and the long-QT syndrome. It is often asymptomatic, but may cause atypical chest pain or palpitations. There is an association with sudden death. Squatting, by increasing afterload increases the intensity of the murmur, the opposite of the effect on the murmur of hypertrophic cardiomyopathy.

Causes of aortic stenosis
- Supravalvular
  - Williams Syndrome
  - Familiar hypercholesteblaemia
- Valvular
  - Calcific degenerative
  - Bicuspid aortic valve
  - Unicommisural valve
- Subvalvular
  - Subvalvular diaphragm
  - Hypertrophic cardiomyopathy

Acquired Valvular Disease

Q 11. Aortic regurgitation may be found in all the following except:

    A. Bicuspid aortic valve
    B. Primary syphilis
    C. Ankylosing spondylitis
    D. Coarctation of the aorta
    E. William's syndrome

Q 12. A 40-year-old woman is admitted to hospital with a fever of 38°C. She had an aortic valve replacement 2 years previously following an episode of bacterial endocarditis. On examination there are needle tracks on her forearms. There are 2 splinter haemorrhages on her left hand and 6 splinters on the right hand. She has mild tenderness in the left upper quadrant of the abdomen. Urine dipstick shows blood +++. ECG shows sinus tachycardia with first degree heart block. Blood cultures are awaited. Which of the following is true?

    A. A history of IV drug abuse would suggest coagulase negative staphylococci as the causative agent
    B. Endocarditis beyond 6 months of surgery is usually due to *Staphylococcus epidermidis*
    C. Daily ECGs are useful in monitoring infections of the aortic valve
    D. Valve surgery should be delayed until the patient is apyrexial
    E. A normal transoesophageal echocardiogram excludes the diagnosis

A 11. B

Chronic aortic regurgitation (AR) can occur with leaflet problems (bicuspid aortic valve, calcific degeneration, William's syndrome), or aortic root problems (seronegative spondyloarthritidies, connective tissue diseases, aortitis). Acute syphilis does not cause an aortitis and is not associated with AR.

A 12. C

Infections of the prosthetic valve beyond 6 months after surgery are most often due to *Streptococcus viridans*. Early infections are usually due to *Staphylococcus epidermidis* (coagulase negative). IV drug abuse may lead to *Staphylococcus aureus* (coagulase positive) infections. One of the major dangers with aortic valve endocarditis is an aortic root abscess. This can lead to prolonging of the PR interval by erosion into the adjacent AV node. Valve surgery may be deferred until the patients is apyrexial unless there is haemodynamic compromise, large vegetations are seen or an abscess present. Note: A normal echocardiogram does not exclude infective endocarditis.

Causes of culture-negative endocarditis
- Wrong diagnosis
- Mycoplasma
- Legionella
- Bartonella
- Q fever
- Brucella
- Fungal
- Marantic
- HACEK group

Causes of aortic regurgitation

	Acute	Chronic
Leaflet	– Infective endocarditis – Rheumatic fever	– Bicuspid valve – Supravalvular aortic stenosis – HOCM – Subaortic VSD

Aortic root	– Dissection
	– Ruptured sinus
	  of valsalva aneurysm
		– Seronegative
		  spondyloarthritides
		– Syphilis (tertiary)
		– Collagen vascular diseases
		– Hypertension

Congenital Heart Disease 1

Q 13. A 28-year-old woman is 23 weeks pregnant and referred for evaluation of a heart murmur. She is asymptomatic. On examination she has triphalangeal thumbs. There is a prominent systolic murmur at the upper left sternal edge. ECG shows right axis deviation, and incomplete RBBB. An echocardiogram shows an ASD. Which of the following statements is true?

    A. There is a recognised association between ASD and triphalangeal thumbs

    B. She should be advised to seek antibiotic prophylaxis for dental procedures

    C. The murmur is produced by associated pulmonary stenosis

    D. She has a low risk of developing pulmonary hypertension now she is an adult

    E. RBBB with a normal axis is the usual ECG finding

Q 14. Ventricular septal defects:

    A. Cause heart failure on the first day of life

    B. Do not require antibiotic prophylaxis if small

    C. Are associated with aortic regurgitation

    D. Are associated with a loud systolic murmur once Eisenmenger's syndrome has occurred

    E. Are associated with lithium exposure in utero

A 13. A

ASDs are the second commonest congenital heart disease seen in adults. They are not benign, with 50% death rate at age 50. Complications rarely occur in childhood, but prolonged shunting leads to pulmonary hypertension, atrial arrhythmias, but not the risk of endocarditis. A Primum defect causes RBBB and LAD, whilst Secundum causes RBBB and RAD on the ECG. The only murmur heard is a pulmonary flow murmur, which is not as pronounced as the murmur of pulmonary stenosis. Secundum ASD is associated with Holt-Oram syndrome, with tri-phalangeal thumb and radial abnormalities.

A 14. C

VSDs are the commonest adult congenital heart disease. They may close spontaneously, and if small cause loud systolic murmurs. This murmur disappears with the onset of Eisenmenger's syndrome as pressures equalise. With high pulmonary artery (PA) pressures at birth, physical signs and the shunt are not pronounced. Heart failure occurs with the lowering of PA pressure after a few weeks. Sub-aortic VSDs are associated with aortic regurgitation. Lithium exposure during development is associated with Ebstein's anomaly.

Congenital Heart Disease 2

Q 15. **Eisenmenger's syndrome:**

  A. May result from Fallot's tetralogy
  B. Is associated with a long PR interval on ECG
  C. Is associated with a systolic murmur if due to VSD
  D. Is associated with patent ductus arteriosus (PDA)
  E. Is treatable with heart transplantation

Q 16. **A 24-year-old woman is referred because her GP noticed a short PR interval and delta wave on a routine ECG. Which of the following is not a recognised association with this condition?**

  A. Hypertrophic cardiomyopathy
  B. Ebstein's anomaly
  C. Mitral valve prolapse
  D. Secundum atrial septal defect
  E. Ventricular tachycardia in the absence of drug therapy

A 15. **D**

Fallot's tetralogy (RVH, pulmonary stenosis, overriding aorta and VSD) causes cyanosis but not pulmonary hypertension. Eisenmenger's syndrome is due to a right to left shunt generated by high pulmonary pressures. The commonest lesions in adult practice to do this are VSD, ASD and PDA. Once the shunt has reversed, the VSD murmur is no longer present, and the only murmur often heard is pulmonary regurgitation. Heart-lung transplantation is required.

A 16. **E**

Wolff-Parkinson-White syndrome (WPW) occurs in 1.5/1000 people. An accessory pathway connects atria to ventricles making the patient prone to atrio-ventricular re-entry tachycardia (AVRT), atrial fibrillation, and atrial flutter. A broad complex tachycardia can result from conduction down the accessory pathway and up the AV node during AVRT, but VT does not occur. AF can degenerate very rapidly to VF as the accessory pathway does not slow conduction, and this is the main cause of death.

Eisenmenger's syndrome
- Reversal of a left to right cardiac shunt due to pulmonary vascular disease caused by increased flow (e.g. VSD, ASD, PDA)
- Complications of
  - Right heart failure
  - Arrhythmias
  - Systemic emboli
  - Hyperviscosity syndrome
  - Gout
  - Endocarditis
  - Haemoptysis
- Treatment
  - Antibiotic proathylaxis
  - Avoid operative procedures
  - May need to venesect
  - Heart-lung transplant

Arrhythmias and Pacing

Q 17. **Which of the following is not a recognised problem with the use of adenosine?**

A. The need for dose reduction in patients on theophylline
B. The need for dose reduction in patients on disopyramide
C. Production of bronchospasm in patients with asthma
D. Production of chest pain even this normal coronary arteries
E. Possible worsening of re-entry tachycardia in Wolff-Parkinson-White syndrome

Q 18. **A 45-year-old banker is admitted to hospital with an acute inferior myocardial infarction. He receives thrombolysis with streptokinase, with partial resolution of his ST segments. However he develops complete heart block. A temporary pacing wire is inserted and he makes an uncomplicated recovery. However he remains in complete heart block, and is pacing dependent. Which of the following statements is true?**

A. Complete heart block for 72 h after a myocardial infarction is an indication for permanent pacing
B. His ECG will resemble LBBB during ventricular pacing
C. Cardiac auscultation during pacing will show widely split second heart sound
D. Complete heart block is best treated with single chamber permanent pacing
E. MRI scanning can be safely performed >3 months after insertion of a permanent pacemaker

A 17. **A**

The action of adenosine is blocked by theophylline, and enhanced by disopyramide. The patient should be warned about chest tightness and dizziness, and a defibrillator should be at hand in case the tachycardia accelerates, as may happen with the Wolff-Parkinson-White syndrome. Adenosine can produce profound bronchospasm and should be avoided in asthmatics.

A 18. **B**

Permanent pacing can be single chamber atrial (e.g. AAI), single chamber ventricular (e.g. VVI) or dual chamber (e.g. DDD). The first letter stands for the sensed chamber, the second for the paced chamber, and the third for what happens to the pacing if a native heart beat is detected (I = inhibited pacing, D = inhibit if ventricular beat sensed, pace ventricle if atrial beat detected). RV pacing makes the ECG look like LBBB. Therefore, A2 is late, and the second heart sound is reversed split. The metal in the pacing box precludes MRI scanning. Strong electrical fields should also be avoided as pacing may be disrupted. After an MI, a permanent pacemaker is usually not inserted for up to 10 days, as most inferior MI's recover conduction, whilst most anterior MI's with CHB die due to the size of the infarct that causes this combination.

WPW is associated with:
- Mitral valve prolapse
- Secundum ASD
- Ebsteins anomaly (WBW-B)
- Thyrotoxicosis
- Hypertrophic cardiomyopathy

Ischaemic Heart Disease

Q 19. The following are absolute contra-indications to thrombolysis for an acute myocardial infarction (MI):

    A. Menstruation finished 2 days previously
    B. Indigestion for 2 years
    C. Proliferative diabetic retinopathy
    D. Ischaemic stroke 18 months previously
    E. Total hip replacement 7 days previously

Q 20. All the following are associated with increased rates of myocardial infarction except:

    A. Haemochromatosis
    B. Systemic Lupus Erythematosis (SLE)
    C. Anti-phospholipid syndrome
    D. Kawasaki disease
    E. Rheumatoid arthritis

A 19. **E**

The contra-indications to thrombolysis have reduced over time. Operation within 10 days, pregnancy, previous subarachnoid haemorrhage, haemorrhagic stroke <1 year prior, active bleeding <10 days before are the only absolute contra-indications. Questions are often asked about dissection etc., and the wrong diagnosis is obvious contra-indications. Proliferative diabetic retinopathy is not an absolute contra-indication, but a 'relative' one.

A 20. **A**

It is now recognised that chronic inflammatory conditions, in particular SLE, can cause accelerated atherosclerosis. Kawasaki disease leads to coronary aneurysms, which can cause MI by related thrombosis or stenosis. MI can also result from coronary thrombosis, predisposed to by anti-phospholipid syndrome. Haemochromatosis can result in a cardiomyopathy, but not MI.

Pericardial Disease

Q 21. A 64-year-old woman is undergoing investigation for breathlessness. All the following would be in keeping with a diagnosis of constrictive pericarditis except:

  A. Elevated JVP with absent y descent
  B. Peripheral oedema
  C. Orthopnoea
  D. Ascites
  E. Previous cardiac surgery

Q 22. Cardiac tamponade may occur with all except:

  A. Tuberculosis
  B. Rheumatic fever
  C. Pneumococcal pneumonia
  D. Rheumatoid arthritis
  E. Uraemia

A 21. **A**

Constriction produces an elevated JVP, with prominent x and y descent. Pulsus paradoxus occurs less frequently than in tamponade. Other signs include oedema, ascites, hepatomegaly, orthopnoea and dyspnoea. Constriction can be a subtle cause of dyspnoea after cardiac surgery.

A 22. **B**

All the above cause pericarditis, but rheumatic fever does not lead to tamponade that needs decompression.

Differentiation – Tamponade from constriction

	Constriction	Tamponade
JVP	Big X and Y descent	Big X no Y descent
Kussmaul Sign	Yes	No
Pulsus paradoxus	No	Yes
Elevation of atrial pressure	Yes	Yes
Dip and plateau ventricular diastolic trace	Yes	No

Blood Vessel Disease

Q 23. **A 35-year-old man presents with 2 h of 'tearing' chest pain. Which of the following factors is most suggestive of a diagnosis of aortic dissection?**

A. Profound vomiting prior to pain
B. History of syphilis
C. Down's syndrome
D. Noonan's syndrome
E. Hypotension

Q 24. **Coarctation of the aorta:**

A. Is more common in women
B. Is associated with rib notching all 12 ribs on the left
C. Is commonly associated with pulmonary stenosis
D. Rarely causes problems in paediatric life
E. Is associated with berry aneurysms

A 23. **B**

Dissection of the aorta is associated with hypertension, cocaine abuse, trauma, pregnancy, and with aortitis as seen in syphilis, SLE. It is also associated with Marfan's and Ehlers-Danlos syndrome. By association with coarctation, it is also associated with Turner's syndrome, but not with Down's syndrome or with Noonan's syndrome. Severe vomiting suggests oesophageal rupture as a cause. Dissection is usually associated with hypertension.

A 24. **E**

Coarctation can cause heart failure in the neonate and hypertension in the adult. It is associated with Turner's syndrome, neurofibromatosis, bicuspid aortic valve, and more weakly with VSD and ASD. Stroke may result from hypertension or from associated berry aneurysms. As with all left heart obstructions, it is more common in males. Notching of ribs 3–8 is seen. Notching or ribs 1 and 2 suggests inferior vena cava obstruction, a Blalock shunt or hypertrophied nerves.

Complications of dissection of the ascending aorta
- Complete tear – Exsanguination
- Forwards tear
  - Stroke
  - Paraplegia
  - Loss of limb pulses
  - Renal failure
- Backwards tear
  - Aortic regurgitation
  - Myocardial infarction
  - Tamponade

Cardiovascular Pharmacology 1

Q 25. The following drugs enhance the effects of warfarin:

A. Phenytoin
B. Rifampicin
C. Carbamazepine
D. Cimetidine
E. Pravastatin

Q 26. Digoxin toxicity is more likely with:

A. Hyperkalaemia
B. Hypocalcaemia
C. Hypomagnesaemia
D. Hyperthyroidism
E. Spironolactone

[A] 25. D

Pravastatin does not interact with warfarin, whereas simvastatin can theoretically raise the INR slightly by inhibiting the metabolism of warfarin. Cimetidine, being a P450 enzyme inhibitor potentiates warfarin greatly. Phenytoin, rifampicin and carbamazepine are enzyme inducers and so reduce the effects of warfarin.

[A] 26. C

Hypomagnesaemia, hypokalaemia, and hypercalcaemia worsen digoxin toxicity. Digoxin overdose can produce hyperkalaemia by inhibiting the Na/K ATPase. Spironolactone has no direct interaction with digoxin, but by raising potassium levels may reduce the chance of digoxin toxicity.

Potentiators of digoxin toxicity
- Electrolytes
  - Hypokalaemia
  - Hypomagnesaemia
  - Hypercalcaemia
- Hypothyroidism
- Hypothermia
- Amyloidosis
- Acute myocardial infarction
- Drugs
  - Amiodarone/warfarin
  - Diltiazem/verapamil
  - Quinidine/propafenone

Cardiovascular Pharmacology 2

Q 27. The following drugs are matched correctly with their action:

A. Digoxin stimulates Na/K ATPase
B. Simvastatin inhibits HMGCoA reductase
C. Sotalol has class I and class III properties
D. Amiodarone shortens the action potential
E. Streptokinase increases fibrinogen levels

Q 28. A 60-year-old diabetic man undergoes an elective coronary angioplasty to relieve a 60% stenosis in his right coronary artery. A 3 mm by 15 mm stent is inserted to produce an optimal angiographic result. Which of the following adjunctive therapies would reduced the risk of restenosis?

A. Angiotensin converting enzyme inhibitors
B. Pravastatin
C. Clopidogrel
D. Low-molecular weight heparin
E. Abciximab in diabetic patients

[A] 27. **B**

Sotalol has class II (β-blocker) and class III (Amiodarone) like actions. Amiodarone prolongs the action potential and the QT interval. Both Sotalol and Amiodarone carry the risk of precipitating ventricular arrhythmias. After thrombolysis, fibrinogen levels are low, due to consumption during thrombosis.

[A] 28. **E**

Restenosis after PTCA is a problem in up to 1/3 of cases. No medication appears to eliminate the risk, but there is some data to suggest that the use of the anti-platelet glycoprotein IIb/IIIa receptor blocker abciximab (ReoPro™) may reduce the risk or restenosis in diabetic patients. The use of stents definitely reduces the rate of restenosis. Clopidogrel reduces acute thrombosis risk, but not restenosis.

Uses of angiotensin converting enzyme inhibitors
- Hypertension
- Heart failure
- Post myocardial infarction
- Patient with risks of vascular disease
- Prevention of diabetic nephropathy
- Treatment of nephrotic syndrome

Other Cardiology

Q 29. A 72-year-old woman is admitted to hospital with sudden onset right arm and leg weakness. She was previously well and independent taking only bendrofluazide for hypertension diagnosed 2 years previously. Examination reveals a right hemiparesis with brisk reflexes and an extensor plantar on the right. She has a soft mid systolic click on auscultation of her chest. There are 5 splinter haemorrhages on her left hand, and she has a cold white left middle finger. CXR shows cardiomegaly and is suggestive of left atrial enlargement. U&Es, FBC and clotting are normal but the ESR is 70 mm/hr. An urgent ECHO reveals a mass in the left atrium. Which of the following clinical features is not explained by this finding?

  A. Embolic CVA on brain CT
  B. The mid-systolic click
  C. Systemic emboli
  D. Left atrial dilatation
  E. Raised ESR

Q 30. In hyperlipidaemia:

  A. Triglycerides (TG) >3 mmol/l give a risk of pancreatitis
  B. Polygenic disorders are more common than monogenic
  C. Statins are the agent of choice in secondary hyperlipidaemia
  D. Lipoprotein lipase (LPL) deficiency elevated LDL more than TG
  E. The liver function tests need to be measured monthly on statin therapy

Myxomas in the heart make up 50% of primary cardiac tumours. They are most common in the left atrium arising from a pedicle on the fossa ovalis. On third present with emboli, a third with systemic inflammation (ESR elevated in 1/3) and a third are asymptomatic when detected. They can intermittently flop through the mitral valve, and cause a mid-diastolic click (tumour plop) when they stop moving. Elevated left atrial pressures cause dilatation. Syncope can occur due to obstruction. They are more common in women.

A triglyceride level >15 mmol/l increases the risk of pancreatitis. Lower levels probably increase coronary risk in association with low HDL levels. Secondary hyperlipidaemias need treatment of their cause (e.g. nephrotic syndrome) as well as treatment of the lipid abnormality. When first marketed, there was concern about both rhabdomyolysis and hepatic dysfunction with statin therapy. Routine measurements of CK or LFT's are not called for. LPL deficiency is a cause of elevated triglycerides more than of cholesterol, but polygenic disorders are much more common than monogenic ones.

Causes of sudden cardiac death
- Arrhythmia
  - Acute myocardial infarction
  - Long-QT syndromes
  - Hypertrophic cardiomyopathy
  - Commotio cardis
  - Coronary anomalies
  - Myocarditis
- Obstruction
  - Atrial myxoma
  - Infective endocarditis
- Dissection

Dermatology

Erythema Nodosum

Q 1. The following are true of erythema nodosum except:

   A. It can present with painful nodular lesions on the arms
   B. Systemic steroids are required as treatment in most cases
   C. Brucellosis is a cause
   D. It is inflammation of the subcutaneous fat
   E. The lesions resolve without scarring

Q 2. A 35-year-old woman presents with tender raised nodules on her shins. Which of the following investigations would not be useful?

   A. Chest X-ray
   B. Serum calcium
   C. Throat swab
   D. X-ray of the lower legs
   E. Anti-streptolysin-O titre

A 1. **B**

A 2. **D**

Erythema nodosum is a reactive inflammation of the subcutaneous fat (a panniculitis). Painful nodules usually occur on the shins, but less commonly on the forearms or thighs, and resolve spontaneously within 6 weeks without scarring. It is important to investigate for an underlying cause. Bed rest and non-steroidal analgesics provide symptomatic relief.

Erythema nodosum
- *Causes:*
  1 – Infections
    - Bacteria, e.g. streptococci, brucellosis, syphilis
    - Mycobacteria, e.g. TB, leprosy
    - Viral
    - Fungal, e.g. coccidiodomycosis
    - Other, e.g. leptospirosis, mycoplasma, coxiella, chlamydia
  2 – Drugs, e.g. sulphonamides, oral contraceptive pill, dapsone, aspirin, codeine
  3 – Systemic disease, e.g. sarcoid, ulcerative colitis, Crohn's, Behcet's, Hodgkin's disease
  4 – Pregnancy

- *Investigations:* Look for cause – e.g. CXR, throat swab, ASO titre, serology, calcium, serum ACE. No cause found in 50%
- *Treatment:* Find and treat cause if possible. Bed rest and non-steroidals for symptom relief. Generally self-limiting over about 6 weeks. Systemic steroids are rarely necessary and should not be given 'blind' in case they exacerbate underlying infection.

Erythema Multiforme

Q 3. The following are true of erythema multiforme except:

A. It is a blistering disease
B. The commonest cause in UK is herpes simplex virus infection
C. Palms and soles are affected
D. C1 esterase inhibitor deficiency causes a hereditary form of the disease
E. Oral contraceptive use is a recognised cause

Q 4. A 56-year-old woman is admitted to hospital with a rash involving the palms of her hands and feet. It appears red, raised and annular. There is no involvement of the trunk. Which of the following drugs is least likely to be the culprit?

A. Carbamazepine
B. Allopurinol
C. Ibuprofen
D. Omeprazole
E. Rifampicin

A 3. **D**

A 4. **D**

Erythema multiforme
- A reaction pattern: target lesions on palms, soles and limbs. Mucosal ulceration (conjunctivae, mouth, genitalia) occurs if severe (known as Stevens Johnson syndrome)

Causes
1 – Idiopathic (50%)
2 – Viral infections
- Herpes simplex
- Viral hepatitis
- EBV
- ORF
- Mumps/polio
- HIV
3 – Other infections
- Mycoplasma
- Psittacosis
- Histoplasma
4 – Connective tissue diseases
5 – Malignancy
- Carcinoma
- Lymphoma
6 – Pregnancy
7 – Others
- Sarcoid
- Pregnancy
8 – Drugs
- Antibiotics: sulphonamides, co-trimoxazole, penicillins, cephalosporins, fluoroquinolones, vancomycin
- Anti-epileptics: carbamazepine
- Non-steroidals: piroxicam, ibuprofen, naproxen, diclofenac, sulindac
- Others: allopurinol, oral contraceptive pill
- Drugs are more likely to cause the more severe variant of erythema multiforme with painful mucosal ulceration

Course: may take up to 3 weeks to resolve. Can be recurrent
Treatment: treat cause. Stop suspected drug. In mild cases, treat symptomatically with anti-histamine to relieve itch and topical steroid to reduce inflammation. In more severe cases good eye and mouth care is required. Maintain fluid balance and look for and treat secondary infection. Long term prophylactic aciclovir may help in recurrent cases.

Internal Malignancy

Q 5. Which of the following cutaneous signs is least likely to be associated with internal malignancy?

    A. Ichthyosis
    B. Urticaria
    C. Hypertrichosis lanuginosa
    D. Acanthosis nigricans
    E. Necrolytic migratory erythema

Q 6. A 60-year-old smoker presents with weight loss and skin and nail changes. Which of the following signs is least likely to suggest the diagnosis of an underlying malignancy?

    A. Erythema gyratum repens
    B. Heliotrope rash on eyelids
    C. Nicotine staining of nails
    D. Migratory thrombophlebitis
    E. Finger clubbing

A 5. B

Urticaria can be caused by drugs, infections or underlying connective tissue disease, but is rarely associated with internal malignancy. The heliotrope rash is a feature of dermatomyositis, a condition known to be associated with underlying malignancy. Longitudinal ridging of the nails may be physiological, or occur with lichen planus, rheumatoid arthritis, old age, peripheral vascular disease or Darier's disease. Lichen planus is only very rarely associated with internal malignancy. Finger clubbing is associated with bronchial carcinoma, mesothelioma and GI lymphoma.

A 6. C

The skin may be affected by internal malignancy in 3 ways
1 – *Direct tumour spread:* commonly from lung, breast, tumour and melanoma; Paget's disease of the breast (underlying adenocarcinoma); cutaneous infiltrates of lymphoma and leukaemia (Sezary Syndrome)
2 – *Genetic syndromes* associated with internal malignancy:
   - Von-Hippel Lindau
   - Neurofibromatosis
   - Gorlin's syndrome
   - Peutz-Jegher's syndrome
   - Wiscott-Aldrich syndrome
   - Tuberous sclerosis
3 – *Paraneoplastic syndromes:*
   - Acanthosis nigricans – gastric carcinoma
   - Acquired ichthyosis – lymphoma, breast cancer, myeloma
   - Erythema gyratum repens – solid tumours, e.g. lung, prostate
   - Acquired hypertrichosis lanuginosa
   - Necrolytic migratory erythema – glucagonoma
   - Migratory thrombophlebitis – pancreatic, stomach and lung carcinoma
   - Dermatomyositis
   - Pemphigoid
   - Tylosis (oesophageal – malignancy)
   - Erythema multiforme
   - Pyoderma gangrenosum (myeloma, lymphoma, leukaemia)

Diabetes

Q 7. A random blood glucose would be a useful first line investigation in all of the following dermatological conditions except:

A. Erythema multiforme
B. Necrobiosis lipoidica
C. Vitiligo
D. Eruptive xanthomata
E. Granuloma annulare

Q 8. A 55-year-old overweight lady with Type II diabetes presents with a 6 cm diameter ulcer on the left medial malleolus. What is the most likely cause of this?

A. Neuropathic ulcer
B. Arterial ulcer
C. Pyoderma gangrenosum
D. Venous ulcer
E. Ulcerated squamous cell carcinoma

A 7. **A**

The target lesions of erythema multiforme can be triggered by a variety of stimuli such as infections and drugs. They are not associated with diabetes mellitus. All the rest are recognised associations or complications of diabetes.

A 8. **D**

Pyoderma gangrenosum is an inflammatory ulcerative condition associated with Crohn's, ulcerative colitis, rheumatoid arthritis and leukaemia. Neuropathic ulcers tend to occur on the feet, and arterial ulcers are more common on the dorsum of the foot, heel, calf and shin. By far the most common type of leg ulcer is venous, and the typical site is on the medial malleolus. The main risk factor for venous ulcers is previous deep vein thrombosis, although perpetuating factors include obesity and hypertension.

Skin conditions occurring in diabetes
- Necrobiosis lipoidica
- Granuloma annulare
- Candidal infections including oral, genital and flexural candidiasis (Intertrigo)
- Staphylococcal infections
- Neuropathic foot ulcers
- Vitiligo
- Eruptive xanthomata
- Signs of atherosclerosis, e.g. ischaemic ulcers, gangrene

Thyroid Disease

Q 9. A 60-year-old lady has recently been found to be hypothyroid. Which of the following features is **not** related to her endocrine disorder?

A. Eczema
B. Coarse scalp hair
C. Xanthomata
D. Facial oedema
E. Hyperhidrosis

Q 10. A thin 40-year-old lady presents with lesions on her shins. She is noted to have sweaty palms and protruding eyes. The skin lesions are most likely to be:

A. Erythema nodosum
B. Erythema ab igne
C. Pyoderma gangrenosum
D. Pretibial myxoedema
E. Necrobiosis lipoidica

A 9. E

The adult hypothyroid patient is usually a female aged between 40 and 70 years. Cutaneous changes occur early and may be insidious. Absence of sweating (anhidrosis) is a feature of hypothyroidism. In addition to skin changes, thyroid dysfunction, hypo- or hyper-, is a cause of generalised pruritus without a rash.

A 10. D

Erythema nodosum is an inflammation of subcutaneous fat caused by infections, drugs or systemic disease such as sarcoid or Crohn's. Erythema ab igne is the reticulate erythema of skin due to prolonged exposure to local heat, e.g. from a hot water bottle or fire. Pyoderma gangrenosum is an inflammatory ulcerative condition associated with Crohn's, ulcerative colitis, rheumatoid arthritis and leukaemia. Necrobiosis lipoidica is associated with diabetes. In pretibial myxoedema, pink or flesh-coloured plaques are seen on the lower shins, usually associated with exophthalmos. They may persist even when the thyroid disease is treated.

Cutaneous features of hypothyroidism
- Pale, cold, scaly and wrinkled skin
- Absence of sweating
- Yellow skin colour
- Puffy oedema of hands, face and eyelids
- Eczema
- Xanthomata
- Coarse sparse scalp hair, loss of lateral eyebrows
- Purpura and ecchymoses
- Generalised pruritus

Cutaneous features of hyperthyroidism
- Increased sweating especially of the palms and soles
- Distal onycholysis
- Thyroid acropachy
- Pretibial myxoedema
- Urticaria
- Diffuse scalp hair thinning
- Diffuse hyperpigmentation (Addisonian-type but sparse buccal mucosa)
- Generalised pruritus

Vasculitis

Q 11. Which of the following is least likely to be associated with a purpuric rash on the legs?

A. Cutaneous amyloid
B. Sarcoidosis
C. Behçet's disease
D. Hepatitis B infection
E. Waldenstrom's macroglobulinaemia

Q 12. An otherwise well 50-year-old male develops a vasculitic skin rash on the legs. Which of the following investigations is it most important to perform?

A. Blood glucose
B. Thyroid function
C. Renal function
D. Anti-nuclear antibody
E. Blood cultures

A 11. B

In primary amyloidosis, petechiae, purpura and bruising may occur spontaneously or after minor trauma, especially around the eyelids and in body flexures, though any part of the body can be involved. Cutaneous sarcoid manifests as lupus pernio, papular, nodular or plaque-like lesions, and it Koebnerises in scars. It is not commonly associated with purpura or vasculitis. Vasculitis typically presents as painful, palpable purpura usually on the legs. Causes of vasculitis are given in the table below.

A 12. C

On diagnosing cutaneous vasculitis, the most important next step would be to look for systemic involvement, in particular, renal involvement, by urinalysis for proteinuria and haematuria. Blood pressure measurement and renal function are also important. After this, a range of screening investigations is usually performed to look for any underlying cause.

Causes of vasculitis

	Granulomatous	Non-granulomatous
Large vessel	Giant cell	Takaysasu
Medium vessel	Buerger's, Churg-Strauss	P.A.N., Kawasaki
Small vessel	Wegener's	▪ Microscopic polyarteritis ▪ Henoch Schonlein ▪ Connective tissue disease ▪ Essential mixed cryoglobulinaemia ▪ Inflammatory bowel disease ▪ Drugs ▪ Paraneoplastic ▪ Infections (endocarditis, hep B, strep)

Generalised Pruritus

Q 13. A 43-year-old woman is referred with widespread pruritus for several months. There is no obvious rash apart from minor excoriations. Which of the following conditions is the least likely cause of this presentation?

A. Acute intermittent porphyria
B. Hyperthyroidism
C. Iron-deficiency anaemia
D. Hodgkin's disease
E. Polycythaemia

Q 14. A 75-year-old woman presents with severe generalised pruritus but no rash. Which of the following investigations is least useful?

A. Chest X-ray
B. Liver chemistry
C. Blood glucose
D. Serum ACE
E. Ferritin

A 13. A

Acute intermittent porphyria has no skin manifestations. It is caused by mutations in the porphobilinogen deaminase gene. Abdominal pain, neuropsychiatric symptoms, and dark urine are features, sometimes triggered by drugs, e.g. oestrogens, griseofulvin and sulphonamides.

A 14. D

Serum ACE is a test for sarcoid. Sarcoidosis causes erythema nodosum. Cutaneous sarcoid manifests as lupus pernio, papular, nodular or plaque-like lesions, and it Koebnerises in scars. It is not generally associated with pruritus without a rash.

Causes of generalised pruritus without a rash
- Liver disease
- Chronic renal failure
- Hypo- or hyperthyroidism
- Iron-deficiency anaemia
- Underlying malignancy especially Hodgkin's disease
- Diabetes
- Neurological disease, e.g. multiple sclerosis, neurofibromatosis
- Senile pruritus – elderly dry skin may be itchy
- Polycythaemia rubra vera

Nail Disease

Q 15. Which of the following is the least likely cause of onycholysis in a 40-year-old woman?

    A. Raynaud's phenomenon
    B. Thyrotoxicosis
    C. Fungal infection
    D. Trauma
    E. Lichen planus

Q 16. The following are true about nail disease in psoriasis except:

    A. Toe nail pitting is a feature
    B. It is associated with arthropathy
    C. It signifies severe skin disease
    D. It is usually symmetrical
    E. Onycholysis can occur

boxed[A] **15. E**

Onycholysis is a separation of the nail plate from the nail bed. It is usually painless. It may be congenital or acquired, with a proportion being idiopathic. Causes relate to trauma, fungal infections, dermatological disorders such as psoriasis, systemic disease such as hyperthyroidism, impaired peripheral circulation such as occurs in Raynaud's and photosensitivity. Lichen planus causes thinning of the nail plate, longitudinal ridging of the nails, and occasionally pterygium formation where the cuticle grows forward and attaches itself to the nail plate.

boxed[A] **16. C**

Psoriasis causes pitting, onycholysis and thickening of the nails (subungual hyperkeratosis), which can affect fingers and toes. Severity of psoriasis does not correlate with nail changes. However, severe nail involvement correlates with the presence of psoriatic arthritis. The symmetry of the nail disease can help distinguish the changes from those of fungal infection, which is usually asymmetrical. It may coexist with fungal nail infection; send nail clippings for mycological examination to confirm. There is no effective treatment.

Causes of onycholysis
- Congenital, e.g. yellow-nail syndrome, hereditary partial onycholysis, congenital ectodermal defect
- Acquired
  - Idiopathic
  - Dermatological disease, e.g. psoriasis, dermatitis
  - Systemic disease, e.g. hyperthyroidism
  - Impaired peripheral circulation, e.g. peripheral vascular disease, Raynaud's
  - Infection – fungal infection
  - Trauma, e.g. overzealous manicure
  - Photoonycholysis associated with photosensitising drugs, e.g. psoralens (PUVA treatment for psoriasis), doxycycline, demeclocycline

Dermatitis Herpetiformis

Q 17. **Which of the following statements about dermatitis herpetiformis is not true?**

A. Pruritus associated with it is severe
B. Patients with G6PD deficiency respond well to dapsone
C. It is associated with gluten-sensitive enteropathy
D. Immunofluorescence tests show IgA and C3 in dermal papillae
E. Skin biopsy of uninvolved skin is useful in making the diagnosis

Q 18. **Dapsone used in the treatment of dermatitis herpetiformis is least likely to cause which of the following side effects:**

A. Agranulocytosis
B. Lichen planus
C. Haemolysis
D. Neuropathy
E. Methaemoglobinaemia

[A] 17. B

[A] 18. B

Dermatitis herpetiformis
- Chronic sub-epidermal blistering disease associated with gluten-sensitive enteropathy
- *Clinical features:*
  - severe itch (worst itch ever)
  - affects knees, buttocks, elbows and scalp
  - intact blisters are rare – broken by scratching, so grouped excoriations seen on examination
- *Investigations:*
  - direct immunofluorescence of a skin biopsy of normal skin shows granular IgG and C3 in deposits in the dermal papillae
  - anti-endomysial antibodies in serum
  - antigen is tissue transglutaminase (not usually measured)
- *Treatment:*
  - dapsone relieves itch almost instantly, and controls disease well
  - gluten-free diet reduces the requirement for dapsone and is said to reduce risk of small bowel lymphoma
  - other treatment options included sulphapyridine, sulphamethoxypyridazine, heparin
  - patients with G6PD deficiency are particularly at risk of haemolytic anaemia, and dapsone should be avoided in this group

Dapsone side effects
- Haemolysis (those with G6PD deficiency are particularly at risk)
- Hepatitis
- Agranulocytosis
- Methaemoglobinaemia
- Peripheral neuropathy

Photosensitivity

Q 19. A 56-year-old man complains of a rash. The distribution is suggestive of photosensitivity. Which of the following drugs is least likely to be the culprit?

    A. Amiodarone
    B. Psoralens
    C. Chlorpropamide
    D. Omeprazole ✓
    E. Bendrofluazide

Q 20. All of the following skin conditions are aggravated by sunlight except:

    A. Discoid lupus erythematosus
    B. Herpes simplex infection
    C. Porphyria cutanea tarda
    D. Pellagra
    E. Scurvy

A 19. D

Drug-induced photosensitivity is an exaggerated sunburn reaction caused by the drug absorbing ultraviolet radiation. Both UVA and UVB are absorbed by most photosensitising drugs. Omeprazole can cause a lichenoid drug eruption, a bullous drug eruption, Stevens Johnson Syndrome or toxic epidermal necrolysis, but photosensitivity is very rare. Ultraviolet light is used therapeutically to treat some conditions such as psoriasis. A careful drug history is required to prevent adverse burning reactions to phototherapy.

A 20. E

Cutaneous (discoid) lupus erythematosus is classically worsened by sunlight, and high factor sun block should be worn all year round. Individuals prone to recurrent herpes simplex (cold sore) can have this triggered by sunlight. In porphyria cutanea tarda, blisters and milia form on sun-exposed sites, especially backs of hands and face. The condition is associated with excessive alcohol intake. Treatment is by sun block, alcohol avoidance, venesection or low dose hydroxychloroquine. Pellagra is vitamin B7 (niacin) deficiency resulting in dermatitis (on sun-exposed sites), diarrhoea and dementia. Scurvy is a vitamin C deficiency resulting in skin haemorrhage and bleeding gums.

Drugs causing photosensitivity
- Amiodarone
- Chlorpropamide
- Nalidixic acid
- Oral contraceptives
- Phenothiazines
- Psoralens
- Quinidine
- Sulphonamides
- Tetracyclines
- Thiazides

Photoaggravated conditions
- Idiopathic photodermatoses, e.g. solar urticaria, polymorphic light eruption, chronic actinic dermatitis
- Herpes simplex
- Rosacea
- Pellagra
- Porphyrias (except acute intermittent)
- Lupus erythematosus
- Darier's disease
- Drug therapy with certain drugs (see above)
- Xeroderma pigmentosum

Conditions helped by sunlight or phototherapy
- Psoriasis
- Atopic dermatitis
- Cutaneous T cell lymphoma (mycosis fungoides)
- Pruritus of renal or liver failure
- Acne

Sebaceous Gland Disorders

Q 21. A 45-year-old woman with facial flushing and eye problems is diagnosed as having rosacea. Which of the following is least likely to be true?

    A. The rash is worse in sunlight
    B. She has blepharitis as a result of rosacea
    C. Alcohol triggers her flushing
    D. Topical steroids are the best treatment for her
    E. Her flushing may be due to menopausal symptoms

Q 22. A 20-year-old female is on isotretinoin therapy for severe cystic acne. All of the following statements are true except:

    A. Her blood androgens are elevated
    B. Her treatment is giving her nosebleeds
    C. She is on the oral contraceptive pill
    D. Her blood lipids may be elevated as a result of her treatment
    E. Her treatment is giving her dry and gritty eyes

A 21. **D**

A 22. **A**

Rosacea
- *Clinical features:*
  - intermittent flushing
  - papules, pustules and telangiectasiae on central face
  - eventual oedema and permanent induration and thickening of the skin
  - the flushing of rosacea may be confused with menopausal symptoms and rarely the carcinoid syndrome
  - more common in women
- *Aggravating factors:*
  - spicy foods
  - hot drinks
  - alcohol
  - sunlight
  - drugs which cause vasodilatation
- *Complications:*
  - rhinophyma of the nose
  - eye problems – conjunctivitis, blepharitis and keratitis
  - chronic facial oedema
- *Course:*
  - relapsing and remitting
  - tends to be progressive unless treated
  - erythema and flushing tends to be persistent and resistant to treatment
- *Treatment:*
  - avoid aggravating factors
  - topical metronidazole gel, oral tetracyclines
  - AVOID topical steroids as they cause severe rebound flare, plastic surgery may help rhinophyma

Acne
- *Pathophysiology:*
  - increased sebum excretion
  - comedogenesis
  - colonisation of the duct with propionibacterium acnes
  - inflammation
  - androgens known to stimulate sebum excretion, but blood levels of androgens generally normal
- *Drug–induced acne:* occurs with steroids, anabolic steroids, gonadotrophins, anti-epileptics, oral contraceptive, lithium, iodides, bromides, isoniazid
- *Treatment:*
  - topical benzoyl peroxide, antibiotics and retinoic acid
  - oral tetracyclines or erythromycin
  - dianette for women
  - isotretinoin for severe nodulocystic or scarring acne
- *Side effects of isotretinoin:*
  - dry eyes and lips
  - nosebleeds
  - teratogenicity in females
  - raised triglycerides
  - low mood
  - hair thinning
  - muscle aches
  - abnormal liver chemistry

Leg Ulceration

Q 23. Leg ulceration is a recognised complication of cell of the following conditions except:

A. Sickle cell anaemia
B. Acute intermittent porphyria
C. Cryoglobulinaemia
D. Calciphylaxis
E. Cholesterol emboli

Q 24. A 65-year-old lady with rheumatoid arthritis develops a painful ulcer on her left shin. Which of the following is least useful as a next step?

A. Examine for splenomegaly
B. Ankle-brachial pressure index
C. Full blood count
D. Swab of ulcer
E. Compression bandaging to left leg

A 23. **B**

Acute intermittent porphyria has no skin manifestations. Abdominal pain, neuropsychiatric symptoms, and dark urine are features, sometimes triggered by drugs, e.g. oestrogens, griseofulvin and sulphonamides. Haematological disorders associated with indolent leg ulceration include sickle cell disease, hereditary spherocytosis, other haemolytic anaemias and polycythaemia. Calciphylaxis is small vessel calcification in end-stage renal failure and hyperparathyroidism. There is livedo reticularis and patchy necrosis of the subcutaneous fat which then ulcerates. Cholesterol embolisation can result in ischaemic ulceration.

A 24. **E**

Felty's syndrome is the triad of rheumatoid arthritis, leukopaenia and splenomegaly. Lymphadenopathy, skin pigmentation and persistent skin ulceration can occur. Pyoderma gangrenosum is a painful skin ulceration which can also occur in rheumatoid disease. Bacteriology and ankle-brachial pressure index measurement may be useful, but it would be unwise to proceed to compression bandaging without establishing the exact nature of the ulcer.

Causes of leg ulceration
- Trauma, e.g. injury, arefact, iatrogenic
- Infections, e.g. TB, deep fungal, 'tropical'
- Bites, e.g. spiders, scorpions, snakes
- Metabolic: diabetes, gout
- Vasculitis, e.g. SLE, rheumatoid, immune complex disease, pyoderma gangrenosum
- Venous, e.g. varicose veins, post deep vein thrombosis
- Arterial, e.g. atherosclerosis, Buerger's, temporal arteritis, polyarteritis
- Haematological, e.g. sickle cell, spherocytosis, polycythaemia, cryoglobulinaemia
- Neuropathic, e.g. diabetes, leprosy, syphilis, syringomyelia, peripheral neuropathy
- Malignant, e.g. squamous cell carcinoma, basal cell carcinoma, Kaposi's sarcoma, melanoma

Causes of ulceration in rheumatoid arthritis
- Ulceration of rheumatoid nodules
- Trauma
- Felty's syndrome
- Vasculitis
- Pyoderma gangrenosum

Bullous Pemphigoid

Q 25. An 80-year-old lady is admitted to hospital with a rash. For the preceeding 3 weeks she has noticed a widespread itchy, blistering rash over her trunk and limbs. On examination there is a widespread bullous erythematous rash with a combination of intact and burst blisters on the torso and back. Which of the following features is not typical of this condition?

- **A.** Itchy eruption
- **B.** Intact blisters on the torso
- **C.** Mouth ulceration and blisters
- **D.** Presentation at the age of 80 years
- **E.** Presence of IgG and C3 on immunofluorescence of a skin biopsy

Q 26. An isolated 5 cm tense blister on the shin of an otherwise well 75-year-old lady is most likely to be due to:

- **A.** Bullous pemphigoid
- **B.** Pemphigus
- **C.** Insect bite reaction
- **D.** Secondary syphilis
- **E.** Herpes simplex infection

A 25. C

Bullous pemphigoid is an autoimmune sub-epidermal blistering disease. It is more common in the elderly, and usually affects the flexures. The mouth is usually spared. Diagnosis can be confirmed by skin biopsy, on which immunofluorescence tests are usually positive for IgG and C3 deposited at the dermoepidermal junction. The blisters are often preceded by a prodrome of an itchy rash.

A 26. C

An intact blister is rare in pemphigus, as the split in the skin is so superficial that blisters rupture easily leaving erosions. Herpes simplex presents as clusters of small vesicles. Insect bite reactions can frequently become bullous, and the leg is a common site for this.

Bullous pemphigoid
- Itchy, tense blisters arising from erythematous or normal skin, especially flexures, mouth spared
- More common in the elderly
- Autoimmune condition, target antigen is hemidesmosomal protein BP 180 and BP 230
- Histology: Sub-epidermal bullae; immunofluorescence shows IgG and C3 at dermoepidermal junction
- Treatment – large doses of oral prednisolone; azathioprine, cyclophosphamide, mycophenolate mofetil can be used as steroid sparing agents

Pemphigus
- Skin and mouth blisters, rupture to form painful erosions
- Can occur at any age
- Autoimmune condition, target antigen is desmosomal proteins (desmogleins 1 and 3)
- Histology: intra-epidermal split; immunofluorescence shows IgG and C3 intraepidermally
- Treatment – large doses of oral prednisolone; azathioprine, cyclophosphamide, mycophenolate mofetil can be used as steroid sparing agents

Causes of bullae
- Physical: cold, heat, friction, oedema
- Insect bites
- Infections: bullous impetigo, bullous tinea pedis
- Drugs: sulphonamides, frusemide, nalidixic acid, non-steroidals can cause pseudoporphyria
- Bullous fixed drug eruptions
- Congenital: epidermolysis bullosa
- Autoimmune: pemphigoid, pemphigus
- Erythema multiforme
- Bullous vasculitis
- Porphyria cutanea tarda

Drug Reactions

Q 27. Drugs which cause a lichen planus-like (lichenoid) drug reaction include all of the following except:

    A. Sulphonamides ✓
    B. Penicillamine
    C. Omeprazole
    D. Pizotifen
    E. Gold

Q 28. A 50-year-old man develops a widespread desquamating rash after starting sulphasalazine for arthritis. Which of the following statements is true?

    A. The rash is caused by staphylococcal exotoxin
    B. His mouth and eyes are likely to be severely affected
    C. Overall mortality is less than 10% ✓
    D. The diagnosis is toxic shock syndrome
    E. It is safe to give him co-trimoxazole in the future

A 27. A

Sulphonamides can cause a blistering skin reaction, Stevens Johnson syndrome or toxic epidermal necrolysis, but they are not associated with lichen planus.

Drugs that cause lichen planus-like (lichenoid) reactions
- Penicillamine
- Proton pump inhibitors, e.g. omeprazole
- Arsenic
- Gold
- Methyldopa
- Mepacrine
- Thiazides
- Beta blockers
- Non-steroidals, e.g. pizotifen
- Dapsone
- Anti-malarials

A 28. C

Toxic epidermal necrolysis
- A life-threatening drug hypersensitivity reaction, severe variant of Stevens Johnson syndrome
- Large areas of the body are involved, usually greater than 30% of the surface area
- Clinical features: mucosal ulceration affecting mouth, eyes and genitalia, widespread painful erythema, with desquamation and sheeting off of the skin
- Drug triggers: sulphonamides, co-trimoxazole, penicillins, cephalosporins, fluoroquinolones, vancomycin
  - Carbamazepine
  - Piroxicam, fenbrufen, ibuprofen, ketoprofen, naproxen, tenoxicam, diclofenac, sulindac
  - Rifampicin, ethambutol
  - Allopurinol
- More common in: HIV, post bone marrow transplant, severe graft versus host disease, lymphoma, leukaemia
- Poor prognosis if sepsis or renal impairment
- Treatment: stop drug, admit, intensive eye, mouth and skin nursing, fluid balance, monitor renal function, watch for sepsis; steroids may worsen outcome, intravenous immunoglobulin may help

Skin Cancer

Q 29. A 70-year-old man has developed a squamous cell carcinoma on his forehead. Which of the following is unlikely to have contributed to this?

    A. He worked in Burma during the war
    B. He had radiotherapy for tinea capitis as a child
    C. He is on ciclosporin
    D. His brother had melanoma
    E. He is a smoker

Q 30. A 35-year-old woman has a mole on her leg which has recently become bigger and darker. Which of the following does not put her in a higher risk group for malignant melanoma?

    A. Her mother had melanoma
    B. She uses sunbeds
    C. She is a smoker
    D. She has less than 10 moles in total on her skin
    E. The mole is on her leg

A 29. **D**

Squamous cell carcinoma
- Rapidly growing ulcerated nodule usually on sun-exposed site (face, ears, back of hands)
- *Causes:*
  - prolonged sun exposure
  - previous radiotherapy
  - smoking – linked to oral and mucous membrane tumours
  - immunosuppression, e.g. transplant recipients
- *Clinical features:*
  - firm, ulcerated nodule
  - surrounding skin shows signs of sun damage, e.g. actinic keratoses lentigines
  - can arise at the base of a cutaneous horn
- *Prognosis:*
  - metastasis likely if
  - mucosal lesion
  - immunosuppressed patient
  - arising in scar ulcer or radiotherapy treated skin
- *Treatment:*
  - excision
  - earlier the better
  - sun-protection advice to those at risk

A 30. **D**

Malignant melanoma
- *Risk factors:*
  - family history of melanoma in first degree relative
  - past history of melanoma
  - numerous naevi or small moles
  - large atypical or dysplastic naevi
  - excessive sun exposure (born or lived in tropics or sub-tropics, e.g. Australia)
  - large numbers of sunburn episodes
  - celtic skin – fair or red hair, blue eyes
- *Clinical features:*
  - lesion showing asymmetry
  - border irregularity
  - colour variability
  - diameter greater than 5 mm
  - elevation irregularity
  - common sites are legs in females and back in males
- *Prognosis:* depends on Breslow thickness, less than 1 mm good prognosis

Breslow (mm)	5 year survival
<1.5	93%
1.5–3.5	67%
>3.5	37%

- *Treatment:*
  - prevention with sun-protection advice, especially children
  - excise all suspected lesions with at least 5 mm clearance margin and check histology

Gastroenterology

Oesophageal Disease 1

Q 1. Which of the following is not a risk factor for the development of oesophageal candidiasis?

A. Diabetes mellitus
B. Inhaled corticosteroid therapy
C. Acquired immunodeficiency syndrome
D. Primary hypogammaglobulinaemia
E. Oral prednisolone therapy

Q 2. A 32-year-old woman presents with recent onset dysphagia to both solids and liquids. Her weight is stable. She had intermittent heartburn during pregnancy but is otherwise symptom free. Her full blood count, urea and electrolytes and liver function tests are all normal. What is the most likely diagnosis?

A. Adenocarcinoma of the oesophagus
B. Squamous cell carcinoma of the oesophagus
C. Oesophageal web secondary to Plummer-Vinson syndrome
D. Achalasia of the oesophagus
E. Peptic stricture of the oesophagus

A 1. **D**

Fungal and yeast infections depend on cell mediated immunity rather than an antibody response. The presence of an increased glucose component in the extracellular fluid provides a useful growth medium for most infective agents.

A 2. **D**

This woman's age and lack of weight loss suggests a benign cause for her dysphagia. The normal full blood count rules out Plummer-Vinson (aka Patterson-Kelly, the presence of an oesophageal web and iron deficiency anaemia). Peptic strictures cause gradual onset dysphagia to solids and then to liquids and would be rare in someone with few reflux symptoms.

Achalasia
- Failure of relaxation of the lower oesophageal sphincter
- Rapid onset dysphagia to both solids and liquids, especially cold food
- The oesophagus is dilated, resulting in pooling of food. Diagnosis: endoscopic features, a barium swallow – the rats tail appearance, and manometry of the sphincter showing its failing to relax
- Treatment options: balloon dilatation, botulinum toxin injections or a laproscopic Heller's myotomy

Causes of dysphagia

Dysmotility:
- Achalasia
- Systemic sclerosis
- Corkscrew oesophagus
- Old age

Strictures:
- Peptic strictures
- Oesophageal webs
- Oesophageal malignancy

Inflammatory:
- Severe oesophagitis (reflux or candidal)

Neurological:
- Cerebrovascular accident

Other:
- Globus hystericus
- Foreign body
- External compression (lymph nodes, malignancy)
- Severe mitral stenosis (Large left atrium pushing into oesophagus)

Gastro-oesophageal Reflux Disease

Q 3. Which of the following is the most effective in the treatment of gastro-oesophageal reflux disease?

A. Ranitidine 300 mg BD
B. Omeprazole 20 mg OD
C. Bismuth TDS
D. Magnesium trisilicate PRN
E. Aluminium hydroxide

Q 4. A 48-year-old woman complains of worsening reflux dyspepsia. Of the following, which would not be implicated in the worsening symptoms?

A. Nifedipine
B. Alcohol
C. Isosorbide mononitrate
D. Domperidone
E. Chewing gum

A 3. **B**

Proton pump inhibitors will control symptoms and heal oesophagitis in 90% within 8 weeks, compared with 40–50% for ranitidine. Additional measures, such as raising the head of the bed, stopping smoking and ethanol intake are important.

A 4. **D**

The worsening symptoms are due to reduced oesophageal sphincter tone that allows reflux. Domperidone is a centrally acting anti-emetic with some pro-kinetic effect, increasing sphincter tone. The others all reduce lower oesophageal sphincter tone. Chewing gum and swallowing saliva would increase symptoms.

Oesophageal Disease 2

Q 5. The following are features of Barrett's oesophagus except:

    A. Small intestinal metaplasia of the normal squamous mucosa
    B. Increased risk of oesophageal adenocarcinoma
    C. Association with gastro-oesophageal reflux disease
    D. The presence of goblet cells
    E. The presence of cuboidal mucosal phenotype

Q 6. A 42-year-old alcoholic is undergoing investigations for dyspepsia. On upper GI endoscopy he is noted to have prominent lower oesophageal varices. Further questioning reveals he has never been admitted to hospital with GI bleeding. Which of the following therapies is least likely to reduce his risk of variceal bleeding in the future?

    A. Propranolol
    B. Variceal sclerotherapy
    C. Variceal banding
    D. Nandolol
    E. Isosorbide mononitrate

A 5.   E

Barrett's oesophagus is the presence of columnar intestinal type mucosa of the small intestinal type replacing the normal squamous mucosa of the oesophagus. There is a small but significant increased risk of adenocarcinoma arising within this metaplasia. The metaplastic mucosa exhibits Paneth cells, goblet cells and a brush border. A history of gastro-oesophageal reflux is associated with Barrett's.

A 6.   B

Non-selective β blockade and ISMN reduce portal pressure and reduce the risk of bleeding, as does banding. Despite it being used, sclerotherapy has not been shown to reduce the risk of bleeding as primary prevention, although may reduce the risk of rebleeding after an index bleed. The mortality of variceal bleeding is 30–50% at each episode.

Malabsorption 1

Q 7. A 48-year-old man underwent a partial gastrectomy for a peptic ulcer. In the future, he is at risk of deficiency of:

A. Folate
B. Iron
C. Thiamine
D. Glucose
E. Nicotinic acid

Q 8. A 48-year-old woman with chronic pancreatitis due to gallstones is noted to have a macrocytic anaemia. What is the most likely cause of the anaemia?

A. Bone marrow dysfunction
B. Hypothyroidism
C. Vitamin B12 deficiency
D. Folate deficiency
E. Hyposplenism

A 7. **B**

Gastric acid is required for the conversion of iron from the ferric to the ferrous form. It is the ferrous form that is absorbed. Even if a partial gastrectomy results in a dumping syndrome, malabsorption is rare.

A 8. **C**

Chronic pancreatitis and insufficiency results in the failure of splitting of dietary B12 from R-binders, a reaction that requires trypsin. This inhibits the binding of intrinsic factor to the Vitamin B12, so it is not absorbed.

Causes of macrocytosis
1 – Physiological
- Pregnancy/neonate
- Reticulocytosis (Bleeding/haemolysis)

2 – Metabolic disease
- Ethanol
- Liver disease
- Myxodema (exclude co-existing B12 deficiency)

3 – Haematological
- Acquired sideroblastic anaemia
- Aplastic anaemia
- PNH
- Cold agglutinins
- Myelodysplasia

4 – Megaloblastic
- B_{12}
- Folate deficiency
- Erythro leukaemia

Helicobacter pylori and the Stomach

Q 9.   A 34-year-old man is referred with dyspepsia. He had triple
       therapy for *Helicobacter pylori* 2 months previously. Which of
       the following is the least useful in determining whether
       therapy was successful?

   A. *H. pylori* serology
   B. ^{13}C urea breath test
   C. Endoscopy and biopsy for histology
   D. Endoscopy and urease test
   E. Stool *H. pylori* antigen

Q 10. The following are true of *H. pylori* except:

   A. Infection suppresses gastrin secretion
   B. It is the cause of >90% of duodenal ulceration
   C. It is associated with gastric adenocarcinoma
   D. Eradication of the infection is curative in gastric MALT
      lymphoma in 80%
   E. It is a Gram negative spiral flagellated organism

A 9. **A**

Serology can remain positive for 6 months to a year after successful eradication of the infection.

A 10. **A**

H. pylori is a spiral-shaped Gram negative, urease producing bacterium. Infection results in a chronic gastritis that, if it involves the body of the stomach, reduces acid secretion resulting in an increased gastrin synthesis. 60% of gastric and 95% of duodenal ulcers are related to *H. pylori*. Mucosa associated lymphoid tissue (MALT) lymphomas result from active infection and 80% regress after successful eradication of the organism.

Malabsorption 2

Q 11. As part of investigations for malabsorption, a woman undergoes small bowel biopsy. Histology shows villous shortening but no plasma cells. Which of the following conditions is the most likely diagnosis?

A. Abetalipoproteinaemia
B. Primary hypogammaglobulinaemia
C. Crohn's disease
D. Salmonella infection
E. Amoebiasis

Q 12. All the following conditions can cause malabsorption. Which one causes malabsorption due to a mucosal defect?

A. Chronic pancreatitis
B. Cystic fibrosis
C. Abetalipoproteinaemia
D. Ulcerative colitis
E. Bacterial overgrowth

A 11. B

A 12. C

Bacterial overgrowth causes steatorrhoea due to bile salt deconjugation and vitamin B12 consumption.
Abetalipoproteinaemia is a failure of synthesis of apoB100 in the liver and apoB48 in enterocytes of the intestinal mucosa resulting in malabsorption of fat-soluble vitamins as a result of a failure of chylomicron synthesis.

Mucosal causes of malabsorption
1 – Coliac disease/sprue
2 – Infections, e.g. TB, giardia, bacterial, Whipple's disease
3 – Enzyme defects
   ■ Failure of digestion
   ■ Failure of absorption

Diagnostic value of small bowel biopsy
1 – Coeliac Disease (villous atrophy, monouclear cells, crypt hypertrophy)
2 – Hypogammaglobulinaemia (villous atrophy, no plasma cells)
3 – Abetalipoproteinaemia (lipid infiltration)
4 – Infections: parasites (*Giardia, Coccidia, Strongyloides*); fungal infection (*Histoplasma, Candida*); Whipple's disease (*T. whippellii*)
5 – Crohn's disease (granulomas)
6 – Lymphoma, α heavy chain disease
7 – Intestinal lymphangiectasia

Causes of villous atrophy
1 – Coeliac disease
2 – Whipple's disease
3 – Giardiasis
4 – Small bowel lymphoma
5 – Infective enteritis in children
6 – True lactose intolerance
7 – Kwashiorkor
8 – Cows milk protein intolerance
9 – Zollinger Ellison syndrome
10 – Vitamin B12 deficiency (pernicious anaemia)

Coeliac Disease

Q 13. Which of the following is recognised to be associated with coeliac disease?

    A. Ulcerative colitis

    B. Smoking

    C. Diabetes insipidus

    D. Auto immune hepatitis

    E. Type II diabetes mellitus

Q 14. A 41-year-old woman is diagnosed as having coeliac disease. Which of these immunological features would be most likely to be found in this lady?

    A. HLA DQ2

    B. HLA B27

    C. Anti-nuclear antibodies

    D. p-ANCA

    E. HLA B8 DR2

A 13. D

A 14. A

HLA DQ2 is seen in 90% of patients with coeliac disease and only 30% of the general population. HLA B8 DR3 is associated with many autoimmune diseases (e.g. Rheumatoid arthritis and SLE) as well as coeliac.

Diseases associated with coeliac disease
1 – Auto-immune disease
- Diabetes mellitus
- Thyroid dysfunction
- Hepatitis

2 – Malignancy
- Oesophageal
- Small bowel
- lymphoma

3 – Other
- Hyposplenism
- Dermatitis herpetiformis
- Trisomy 21
- IgA deficiency
- Collagenous colitis

Complications of coeliac disease
1 – Malabsorption
2 – Iron deficiency anaemia (present in 50% at present)
3 – Hyposplenism (Howell Jolly bodies in RBCs)
4 – Hyperparathyroidism (Vitamin D deficiency)
5 – Loss of sex hormone function
6 – Small bowel lymphoma
7 – Oesophageal carcinoma
8 – Infections with capsulated organisms

Endocrine Malignancy of the GI Tract

Q 15. A man is undergoing investigations for recurrent peptic
ulceration. Serum gastrin levels are elevated, even in the
absence of a proton-pump inhibitor. A gastrinoma is suspected.
Which of the following statements is incorrect?

    A. The majority arise in the pancreas
    B. The majority are associated with MEN type II
    C. The majority are malignant
    D. They are associated with B12 deficiency
    E. They are associated with an elevated calcium

Q 16. A 52-year-old woman is referred for non-specific
malaise and lethargy. She has had carcinoid syndrome
diagnosed 3 years previously and is receiving
treatment with octreotide. Which of the following
features is not a manifestation of her carcinoid syndrome?

    A. Systolic murmur over the pulmonary area of the
       precordium
    B. Erythematous thick skin over her shins and legs
    C. Hypotension
    D. Bronchospasm
    E. Diarrhoea

A 15. **B**

All gastrinomas are malignant, however they are slow growing
and metastasize late. The majority occur in the head of the
pancreas. However they may occur in the duodenal wall or the
gastric antrum. The tumour presents due to its neuroendocrine
cell type, with hypergastrinaemia and hyperchlorhydria. The
prolific gastric acid synthesis results in marked gastro-duodenal
ulceration with multiple duodenal ulcers seen at endoscopy.
Diagnosis is based on a high fasting serum gastrin off proton
pump inhibitors and the localisation of the primary tumour by
CT scanning or rarely venous sampling. Gastrinomas are
associated with MEN type I in 25% of cases. The elevated gastrin
and hyperchlorhydria results in vitamin B12 destruction leading
to malabsorption. Treatment involves resection of the primary if
possible and high dose PPI therapy to control symptoms.

A 16. **C**

Carcinoids synthesise and secrete serotonin from
5-hydroxytryptophan and thus may induce nicotinic acid
deficiency (pellagra) leading to diarrhoea, dementia and
dermatitis. Non-metastatic tumours do not cause symptoms as
the liver metabolises the secreted active substances. After
metastasis, the serotonin, histamine and bradykinin result in
cardiac valve lesions, wheeze, flushing and diarrhoea. Diagnosis
is by urinary 5-hydroxyindole acetic acid and octreotide scanning.
However as the tumour is rarely symptomatic prior to metastasis,
it presents late. Octreotide (a somatostatin analogue) is used to
combat symptoms.

Multiple Endocrine Neoplasias

MEN I
- Parathyroid (95%)
  - Adenoma
  - Hyperplasia
- Pituitary (70%)
  - Prolactinoma
  - Growth hormone
  - ACTH
- Pancreas (50%)
  - Islet cell
  - Gastrinoma
  - Vipoma
- Adrenal (40%)
- Thyroid (20%)

MEN IIa
- Adrenal (95%)
  - Phaeochromocytoma
  - Cushings
- Thyroid (70%)
  - Medullary carcinoma
- Parathyroid (60%)
  - Hyperplasia

MEN IIb
- As IIa plus:
  - Marfanoid
  - Ganglioneromas

Infections of the Colon

Q 17. Which one of the following infectious agents may result in toxic megacolon?

    A. *Yersinia* infection
    B. *Clostridium difficile* infection
    C. *Salmonella enteritis*
    D. *Giardia lamblia* infection
    E. Rotavirus

Q 18. Which of the following is **not** true of *Giardia lamblia* infection?

    A. It is a cause of dysentery
    B. It is a cause of steatorrhoea
    C. It is a cause of villous atrophy
    D. It is best treated with metronidazole
    E. It is diagnosed on stool culture

A 17. C

Infection with Campylobacter can also lead to toxic megacolon.

A 18. A

Giardiasis is an infection of the small intestinal mucosa that produces cramping abdominal pain, diarrhoea and malabsorption. Diagnosis is by microscopy of stool or duodenal aspirate/biopsy showing the owl like organism. Treatment is with metronidazole, mepacrine or albendazole.

Predispositions to Giardiasis
1 – ↓ Mucosal immunity
- Hypogammaglobulinaemia
- Selective IgA deficiency
- Coeliac disease
2 – ↓ Stomach acid
- Achlorhydria
- Partial gastrectomy
- PPI's
3 – Others
- Chronic pancreatitis
- Poor hygiene/oral contamination

Causes of toxic megacolon
1 – Inflammatory bowel disease
2 – Amoebic dysentry
3 – Shigella
4 – Salmonella
5 – Campylobacter

Inflammatory Bowel Disease

Q 19. **Which of the following agents is not appropriate for trying to maintain remission in Crohn's disease?**

    A. Mesalazine
    B. Budesonide
    C. 6-mercaptopurine
    D. Anti-TNFα antibodies
    E. Azathioprine

Q 20. **A 38-year-old women with Crohn's disease for 3 years undergoes a small bowel follow through. Which of the following radiological findings would you *not* expect to find?**

    A. Rosethorn ulcers
    B. String sign of Kantor
    C. Smoothly narrowed colon
    D. Skip lesions
    E. Caecal spasm (Stirlin's sign)

A 19. **D**

Infliximab (anti-TNFα antibodies) can induce remission in resistant or fistulating Crohn's disease, but the remission is not maintained. 6-mercaptopurine is the active metabolite of azathioprine.

A 20. **C**

A smooth, narrow colon suggests ulcerative colitis. Crohn's disease can, however, affect all parts of the GI tract.

Extra intestinal manifestations of inflammatory bowel disease
1 – Arthritis
- symmetrical small joint arthritis
- large joint arthritis
- spondylitis and sacroiliitis

2 – Skin
- pyoderma gangrenosum
- erythema nodosum
- enterocutaneous fistula

3 – Eyes
- conjunctivitis
- iritis
- episeleritis

4 – Blood
- macrocytosis (B12 and folate deficiency)
- microcytosis (iron deficiency)
- thrombocythaemia

Skin Manifestations of Hepatitis

Q 21. A 30-year-old intravenous drug abuser with skin lesions is found to have Hepatitis C infection. Which of the following skin conditions is he least likely to have:

    A. Cryoglobulinaemia
    B. Erythema multiforme
    C. Vasculitis
    D. Skin abscess
    E. Erythema chronicum migrans

Q 22. After taking ampicillin for a fever and sore throat for 2 days, a 25-year-old man develops a widespread rash, lymphadenopathy and looks jaundiced. Which of the following is least likely to be associated with his condition?

    A. Atypical T lymphocytes
    B. Positive monospot test
    C. Haemolytic anaemia
    D. Cytomegalovirus infection
    E. Splenomegaly

A 21. **E**

With or without endocarditis, cryoglobulinaemia, vasculitis and erythema multiforme can occur. In hepatitis C associated with intravenous drug abuse. Skin abscesses and ulcers may be seen in intravenous drug abusers, at injection sites. Erythema chronicum migrans is a slowly enlarging annular ring which classically occurs in Lyme disease.

A 22. **D**

Infectious mononucleosis can present with fever, sore throat, lymphadenopathy, splenomegaly, hepatitis and haemolytic anaemia. A widespread macular rash occurs after ampicillin, but this does not indicate lifelong ampicillin allergy. Atypical mononuclear cells are seen in the blood film. The heterophil antibody monospot or Paul-Bunnell test is positive.

Rashes associated with viral hepatitis
- Erythema multiforme (hep C)
- Cryoglobulinaemia (hep C)
- Vasculitis (hep B or C)
- Gianotti-Crosti syndrome – rash on limb extremities in children, self-limiting (hep B)
- Polyarteritis nodosa (hep B)
- Pseudoporphyria – clinically indistinguishable from porphyria cutanea tarda (hep C)
- Lichen planus (hep C)
- Urticaria (hep B or C)
- Erythema nodosum (hep C)
- Autoimmune thrombocytopaenic purpura (hep C)

Infectious mononucleosis
- Epstein-Barr virus infection
- Clinical features: fever, sore throat, lymphadenopathy, splenomegaly, hepatitis and haemolytic anaemia
- Skin manifestations: widespread macular rash, especially after ampicillin
- Investigations: blood film shows atypical lymphocytes; monospot test positive, EBV-specific antibody titres
- Treatment: bed rest, consider oral steroids

Jaundice

Q 23. A 45-year-old man is referred with jaundice. His liver function tests reveal:

Bilirubin	74
ALT	23
AST	30
Alkaline phosphatase	92
γ GT	32
Prothrombin time	12 seconds
Albumin	41 g/L

What is the most likely diagnosis?
A. Crigler Najjar type I
B. Alcohol abuse
C. Hepatitis A
D. Gilberts syndrome
E. Wilson's disease

Q 24. In which of the following is the defect found in Dubin-Johnson Syndrome?

A. Glucuronysyl transferase
B. Canilicular multispecific organic anion transporter (cMOAT)
C. Stellate cell CD4 receptors
D. Hepatic alkaline phosphatase
E. Melanin synthesis

A 23. D

The diagnosis of Gilberts is based on a bilirubin of <102 mmol/l and otherwise normal liver function. Patients with Crigler-Najjar type I do not survive to adulthood, whereas those with type II do. Both syndromes are due to defects in the glucuronosyl transferase enzyme complex, responsible for the conjugation of bilirubin.

A 24. B

This is a membrane transport complex. Abnormalities result in reduced melanin and bilirubin transport out of the hepatocyte, leading to a conjugated hyperbilirubinaemia and melanin deposition → black liver.

Hepatitis B Infection

Q 25. **Which of the following is true of hepatitis B serology?**

    A. HB e antibodies are a marker of infectivity

    B. HB surface antigen positivity suggests adequate immunisation

    C. HB core IgG antibodies suggest chronic infection

    D. Pre core mutants are characterised by positive HBe antigen and negative HB surface antigen.

    E. HB surface antigen is the first serological marker of infection

Q 26. **Which of the following is true of chronic hepatitis B?**

    A. It follows 30% of all acute hepatitis B infection

    B. It is characterised by HBs antibody positivity

    C. It is often associated with a normal bilirubin

    D. It involves incorporation of hepatits B RNA into the hepatocyte genome

    E. Does not occur in the presence of the Delta virus

A 25. E

HBs Antigen	first marker of infection
HBe Antigen	second marker of infection and infectivity if persistant
HBs antibody	immunity due to exposure or immunisation
HBe antibody	seroconversion
HBc antibody	IgM acute infection or chronic hepatitis (low titre) IgG past exposure
HBV DNA	measure of the viral load
Pre core mutants	are unable to synthesize HBe antigen but are HBs antigen positive in the acute phase

A 26. C

Of all HB infection, 10% → chronic infection of which 10–30% → chronic hepatitis. Patients are usually HBe antigen positive, HBs antigen positive and HBe antibody negative with high HBV DNA initially (the replicative phase). The viral DNA gets incorporated into the hepatocytes and often HBe antigen disappears. Cirrhosis and hepatocellular carcinoma are increased in this group.

Liver Disease and Cirrhosis

Q 27. **The following are histological features of liver cirrhosis on a liver biopsy except:**

   A. Nodular regeneration
   B. Fibrous septa formation
   C. Liver cell necrosis
   D. Granuloma formation
   E. Subendothelial fibrosis

Q 28. **The following are all causes of liver cirrhosis except:**

   A. Galactosaemia
   B. Veno-occlusive disease
   C. Methotrexate
   D. Schistosomiasis
   E. Wilson's disease

A 27. D

The rest represent the classical changes. Micronodular cirrhosis produces nodules that are less than 3 mm across with uniform liver involvement. They are seen in alcoholic liver disease or biliary disease. Macronodular cirrhosis produces larger nodules, and is classically seen in chronic viral hepatitis.

A 28. D

Schistosomiasis causes portal hypertension and periportal fibrosis but not cirrhosis. Indeed, liver function remains remarkably good in chronic infection.

Causes of Hepatic Cirrhosis
- Alcohol
- Hepatitis B +/− D
- Hepatitis C

Autoimmune:
- Primary and secondary biliary cirrhosis
- Autoimmune hepatitis

Inherited/congential:
- Hereditary haemochromatosis
- Wilson's Disease
- α_1 anti-trypsin deficiency
- Galactosaemia
- Glycogen storage disease
- Cystic fibrosis

Vascular:
- Hepatic venous congestion
- Budd-Chiari syndrome
- Veno-occlusive disease

Other:
- Intestinal bypass operations for obesity

Biliary Disease

Q 29. A 68-year-old man presents with jaundice, weight loss and pruritis. He has dark urine and clay like stools. Fasting abdominal ultrasound reveals an empty gallbladder, and intrahepatic duct dilatation. What is the most likely diagnosis?

A. Carcinoma of the head of the pancreas
B. Gastrinoma of the head of the pancreas
C. Cystic duct gall stone impaction
D. Cholangiocarcinoma of the left main bile duct
E. Lymphadenopathy at the porta hepatis

Q 30. Which of the following increases the risk of gallstones?

A. Ileal resection for Crohn's disease
B. Partial gastrectomy for a gastric ulcer
C. Left hemicolectomy for sigmoid carcinoma
D. Left lobectomy of the liver for carcinoid
E. Jejunal resection of gastrointestinal lymphoma

A 29. E

This question requires knowledge of anatomy. For the gallbladder to be empty, the obstruction must be higher than the point of entry of the cystic duct to the common bile duct. For there to be left and right intrahepatic duct dilatation, the obstruction must be at or below the bifurcation of the left and right bile ducts. Therefore only E could cause the findings.

A 30. A

Ileal resection reduces the reabsorption of bile salts and as a result, a reduction in the enterohepatic circulation of bile salts. This increases the risk of cholesterol stones forming.

Haematology

Macrocytosis

Q 1. An 80-year-old woman presents with an MCV of 102 fl. Which of these is the least likely cause of this abnormality?

A. Myelodysplastic syndrome
B. Myeloma
C. Azathioprine treatment for Rheumatoid Arthritis
D. Hyperthyroidism
E. Folate deficiency

Q 2. A 65-year-old woman presents with the following full blood count. Hb 9.3 g/dl, MCV 115 fl, WBC 3.8 × 10^9/l, platelets 120 × 10^9/l. What is the most likely diagnosis?

A. Alcohol abuse
B. Aplastic anaemia
C. Pernicious anaemia
D. Myeloma
E. Hepatitis

A 1.   D

Hyperthyroidism is not associated with a macrocytosis, but may be associated with a neutrophilia, lymphocytosis, neutropenia, thrombocytopenia and occasionally a pancytopenia. B12 deficiency and folate deficiency are the only common causes of an MCV over 110fl.

A 2.   C

Pernicious anaemia is an auto immune cause of B12 deficiency and may cause a pancytopenia with a marked macrocytosis. Alcohol abuse, aplastic anaemia and myeloma could all cause pancytopenia but usually only with a slight increase in MCV. Hepatitis may rarely cause aplastic anaemia, but such a marked macrocytosis would not be seen.

Causes of macrocytosis
Megaloblastic
- B12 and folate deficiency
- Anti folate drugs – methotrexate, pentamidine, trimethoprim
- Drugs interfering with DNA synthesis – azathioprine, cyclophosphamide, hydroxyurea
- Rare inherited defects of DNA synthesis
- Erythro-leukaemia

Others
- Myelodysplastic syndrome
- Myeloma
- Alcohol
- Liver disease
- Phenytoin
- Hypothyroidism
- Diamond-Blackfan anaemia
- Aplastic anaemia
- Down's syndrome
- COAD
- Pregnancy
- Paroxysmal nocturnal haemoglobinuria

Associated with reticulocytosis – Haemolytic anaemia, haemorrhage

Thrombocytopenia

Q 3. You are asked to see a 73-year-old man with a platelet count of $80 \times 10^9/l$ who has been admitted to the CCU with a possible acute coronary syndrome. This is his first presentation with chest pain. Past history includes chronic lymphatic leukaemia diagnosed 8 years ago. 5 years ago he was involved in a traffic accident and required emergency splenectomy. He has had hypertension for the past 3 years treated with bendrofluazide. On examination he is pain free and comfortable. He looks a little malnourished. There is no purpura. He is receiving intravenous unfractionated heparin. Which of the following is least likely to be the cause of the thrombocytopenia?

- A. B12 deficiency
- B. Thiazide diuretic therapy
- C. Chronic lymphocytic leukaemia
- D. Heparin therapy
- E. Splenectomy 5 years previously

Q 4. Which of the following statements about disseminated intravascular coagulation (DIC) is true? Disseminated intravascular coagulation is:

- A. Most commonly associated with Gram positive septicaemia
- B. Commonly associated with a raised fibrinogen level
- C. A frequent presentation of acute myelomonocytic leukaemia (AML M4 subtype)
- D. Usually associated with raised D-dimers
- E. Associated with microthrombotic lesions such as gangrene of digits in over 30% of cases

A 3.   **E**

B12 deficiency can cause an isolated thrombocytopenia or pancytopenia. Thrombocytopenia may also be caused by treatment with thiazide diuretics and heparin. Chronic lymphatic leukaemia may cause thrombocytopenia due to marrow infiltration or due to auto immune thrombocytopenia. Following a splenectomy, patients tend to have a thrombocytosis, which may be as high as $1000 \times 10^9/l$, due to redistribution of platelets.

A 4.   **D**

DIC is associated with septicaemia in 60% of cases, but this is usually due to Gram negative organisms. It may also be associated with acute promyelocytic leukaemia (AML M3). It is associated with microthrombotic lesions in 5–10% of cases, and is usually associated with hypofibrinogenaemia and raised D-dimers and FDPs. These may not be raised in severe DIC due to irreversible organ failure and this confers a poor prognosis.

Causes of thrombocytopenia

Congenital
- May-Hegglin anomaly, Bernard Soulier syndrome, TAR syndrome (Thrombocytopenia with absent radii), Fanconi's anaemia

Acquired
- Drugs – thiazide diuretics, interferon
- Myelodysplastic syndrome
- Paroxysmal nocturnal haemoglobinuria
- Alcohol abuse
- Rarely – severe iron deficiency, parvovirus infection
- Increased platelet consumption or destruction

Immune mechanisms
- Congenital – neonatal alloimmune thrombocytopenia, transplacental transfer of maternal antibody
- Autoimmune thrombocytopenia (AITP) – idiopathic, secondary to autoimmune disease or lymphoproliferative disorders (Chronic lymphocytic leukaemia, Non Hodgkin's or Hodgkin's lymphoma)
- Drug induced – including heparin induced thrombocytopenia
- Post infection – rubella, chicken pox, infectious mononucleosis
- AITP associated with HIV (presenting complaint, not poor prognostic factor)
- Post transfusion purpura

Non-immune mechanisms
- Disseminated intravascular coagulation
- Thrombotic thrombocytopenia purpura
- Infections – viral haemorrhagic fevers, dengue fever, malaria
- Massive transfusion

Other mechanism/mechanism unknown
- Hypersplenism (due to redistribution of platelets – platelet pooling)
- Hypothermia
- Wiskott-Aldrich syndrome, Chediak Higashi syndrome
- Congenital infections – toxoplasmosis, CMV, rubella
- Grave's disease
- Pregnancy (dilutional)
- Paracetamol overdose

Iron Metabolism

Q 5. A 50-year-old man presents with a haemoglobin of 7.6 g/dl and a MCV of 72 fl. Which of the following investigations would be most in keeping with a diagnosis of iron deficiency anaemia?

A. A reduced total serum total iron binding capacity
B. A serum ferritin in the low normal range
C. An increased level of soluble transferrin receptors
D. An increased transferrin saturation
E. A normal serum iron level

Q 6. A 45-year-old man with haemochromatosis comes to your clinic with his wife. They have a number of questions for you. Which of the following statements is true?

A. It is an autosomal dominant condition and so his children should be screened
B. There is an increased risk of autoimmune endocrine diseases such as hypothyroidism
C. It causes hepatocellular carcinoma in over 80% of established cases
D. It can be screened for with a simple blood test in the majority of patients
E. Treatment with phlebotomy can reverse all clinical manifestations

A 5. C

Iron deficiency is associated with an increased level of soluble transferrin receptors. A ferritin level in the lower end of the normal range would not exclude iron deficiency if there is co-existent disease as ferritin is an acute phase protein and will increase in infection, inflammation and malignancy. Serum iron is influenced by recent oral intake and can be normal in an iron-deficient patient who has recently had a high oral iron intake.

A 6. D

The common mutations causing genetic haemochromatosis can now be screened for with a straight forward PCR (polymerase chain reaction) test which is widely available.

Iron deficiency
- Meat and liver are better sources of dietary iron than vegetables, eggs or dairy foods
- Dietary iron is partially absorbed as haem and partly broken down in the gut to inorganic iron
- Absorption occurs in the duodenum and is increased by acid (including vitamin C) and in iron deficiency. Absorption is decreased by alkalis, tea (tannins), bran and iron overload
- Causes of iron deficiency are blood loss, increased demands, malabsorption and poor diet
- Investigations show a hypochromic microcytic anaemia

	Serum iron	Serum ferritin	Marrow iron	Serum TIBC	Transferrin saturation	Transferrin receptors
Iron deficiency	reduced	reduced	reduced	increased	reduced	increased
Anaemia of chronic disorders	reduced	normal/ increased	normal/ increased	reduced	reduced	normal

- Treatment is usually with 200 mg oral ferrous sulphate three times a day. Intramuscular or intravenous iron preparations may be used in certain circumstances

Genetic haemochromatosis
- Autosomal recessive condition
- Associated with an abnormality in HFE gene on chromosome 6
- 80% have missense mutation C282Y and 15% have H63D mutation, which can both be screened for with PCR methods
- 25% of patients with established haemochromatosis and cirrhosis will develop hepatocellular carcinoma
- Other complications are diabetes, skin pigmentation and joint problems
- Phlebotomy is treatment of choice and if initiated before onset of complications and maintained can prevent development of all complications and patient will have normal life expectancy

Sickle Cell Anaemia

Q 7. A patient with sickle cell anaemia presents with a full blood count showing Hb 3.3 g.dl and a reticulocyte count of 0.1%. What is the most likely diagnosis?

A. Severe vaso-occlusive crisis
B. Splenic sequestration
C. Gastro-intestinal haemorrhage
D. Parvovirus infection
E. Sickle chest crisis

Q 8. In the ante-natal clinic a woman is found to have a normal haemoglobin and MCV, but the screening test for sickle haemoglobin is positive and haemoglobin electrophoresis shows HbA 55% and HbS 45%. Her partner has a microcytic anaemia and haemoglobin electrophoresis shows a HbA band only with HbA$_2$ quantitation of 4.8%. What is the least likely haematological diagnosis in the fetus?

A. Sickle cell trait
B. Haematologically normal
C. B thalassaemia trait
D. Sickle-B thalassaemia
E. Sickle cell anaemia

A 7. D

Parvovirus selectively attacks red cell precursors and in anyone with a haemolytic anaemia and shortened red cell survival will cause profound anaemia with a very low reticulocyte count. The other complications of sickle cell disease listed will all cause anaemia, but will be associated with a raised reticulocyte count and will have characteristic clinical signs. A vaso-occlusive crisis is associated with bony pain and sickle chest crisis with shortness of breath and hypoxia. Splenic sequestration occurs in children with sickle cell disease and is characterized by a very rapid enlargement in spleen size as all of the blood volume pools there.

A 8. E

The mother has sickle cell trait (HbAS) and the father has B thalassaemia trait (because of the raised HbA_2). The fetus has a 1 in 4 chance of being haematologically normal (HbAA), having sickle cell trait (HbAS), having B thalassaemia trait and having sickle-B thalassaemia. The latter is a sickling syndrome which can be as severe as homozygous sickle cell disease. If the partner is the father of the child, the child cannot have sickle cell anaemia (HbSS) as the father does not have the sickle gene.

Sickle cell anaemia
- Autosomal recessive condition, glutamine to valine substitution at position 6 on the beta globin chain (chromosome 11)
- HbS will polymerise at low oxygen tensions and causes red cells to irreversibly sickle which results in blockage of the microcirculation
- Clinically painful vaso-occlusive crises are the most common manifestation
- Other features are chest crises, stroke, priapism, splenic and hepatic sequestrations, leg ulcers, cholecystitis, sickle nephropathy, mesenteric sickling, avascular necrosis and retinopathy
- Diagnosis is by haemoglobin electrophoresis, isoelectric focussing or high pressure liquid chromatography (HPLC). PCR methods are used for prenatal diagnosis. The sickle solubility test is positive in heterozygotes (sickle trait) and homozygotes
- Treatment options include transfusion regimes, hydroxyurea and bone marrow transplant

Intravascular Haemolysis

Q 9. A 65-year-old man has recently been started on a tablet to control his hypertension. He presents with a haemoglobin of 9.6 g/dl, MCV 102 fl and polychromasia and spherocytes on his blood film. What is the most likely diagnosis?

    A. Idiopathic auto-immune haemolytic anaemia

    B. Drug induced haemolysis due to underlying glucose-6-dehydrogenase deficiency

    C. Hereditary spherocytosis

    D. Drug induced haemolytic anaemia

    E. Folate deficiency

Q 10. Which of the following causes intravascular haemolysis?

    A. Hereditary spherocytosis

    B. Warm auto-immune haemolytic anaemia

    C. ABO incompatible blood transfusion

    D. Pyruvate kinase deficiency

    E. Sickle cell disease

A 9. **D**

Methyldopa is an anti-hypertensive agent which commonly causes auto-immune haemolytic anaemia, and as there is a history of recent introduction of a new anti-hypertensive agent, this must be high on the list of differential diagnosis. 60–80% of patients treated with methyldopa will develop a positive Direct Coomb's test and 5–10% will develop overt haemolysis. Other drugs which can cause an auto-immune haemolytic anaemia include mefenamic acid, L-dopa and fludarabine. Idiopathic auto-immune haemolytic anaemia would give a similar clinical picture with macrocytic anaemia, polychromasia, spherocytes and positive Direct Coomb's test. Hereditary spherocytosis would fit the clinical details given, but it would be unusual for this to present at this age. Folate deficiency may occur in any patient with increased red cell turnover, including haemolysis, but on its own would not cause a spherocytic anaemia.

A 10. **C**

Causes of intravascular haemolysis include mismatched blood transfusion (usually ABO). Sickle Cell Disease leads to vascular occlusion rather than intra-vascular haemolysis.

Causes of intravascular haemolysis
- Mismatched blood transfusion (usually ABO)
- G6PD deficiency with oxidant stress
- Red cell fragmentation syndromes
- Cold auto-immune haemolytic anaemia
- Some drug and infection induced haemolytic anaemias
- Paroxysmal nocturnal haemoglobinuria
- March haemoglobinuria
- Unstable haemoglobins

Laboratory features of intravascular haemolysis
- Red cells are broken down directly within circulation
- Free haemoglobin rapidly saturates plasma haptoglobins (so haptoglobin levels are low) and excess free haemoglobin is filtered by the glomerulus. Free haemoglobin may enter the urine
- Haemoglobinaemia and haemoglobinuria
- Haemosiderinuira (iron storage protein detected in a spun sample of urine)
- Methaemalbuminaemia (detected spectrophotometrically by Schumm's test)

Causes of spherocytosis
- Hereditary spherocytosis
- Auto-immune haemolytic anaemia

Causes of haemolysis with G6PD deficiency
- Anti-malarials
- Antibiotics (septrin, ciprofloxarin)

Clotting Disorders

Q 11. A 5-year-old girl bleeds excessively after tonsillectomy.
Investigations reveal a normal platelet count and normal PT but
a prolonged APTT. What is the most likely cause?

A. Haemophilia A (factor VIII deficiency)
B. Haemophilia B (factor IX deficiency)
C. von Willebrand's disease
D. Factor XII deficiency
E. Factor V deficiency

Q 12. A patient on the intensive care unit is found to have a
prolonged prothrombin time (PT). Which of these is least likely
to be the cause?

A. Disseminated intravascular coagulation
B. Prolonged antibiotic therapy
C. Massive blood transfusion
D. Acquired factor XII deficiency
E. Liver disease

A 11. C

Von Willebrand's disease is the most common inherited clotting disorder, it causes a prolonged APTT and is usually inherited in an autosomal dominant fashion. Haemophilia A and B will both cause prolongation of the APTT but are both less common than von Willebrand's disease and are both inherited in a X-linked recessive manner, so are very rare in females. Factor XII deficiency will cause a prolongation of the APTT but is not associated with increased bleeding. Factor V deficiency is associated with a prolongation of the PT and the APTT and is extremely rare.

A 12. D

A, B, C and E may all cause prolongation of the PT in the ITU setting. Prolonged antibiotic therapy can lead to Vitamin K deficiency and hence clotting problems. Acquired factor XII deficiency may be seen in sick patients on the ITU, but will cause a prolongation of APTT, not PT.

Clotting cascade
Intrinsic pathway – increased APTT (factors VIII, IX, XI, XII)
Extrinsic pathway – increased PT (factor VII)
Common pathway – increased APTT and PT (factors X, V, II)
Vitamin K dependent factors – II, VII, IX, X

Common causes of a prolonged APTT
- DIC
- Liver disease
- Massive transfusion of stored blood
- Administration of heparin or contamination with heparin
- Deficiency of a coagulation factor other than factor VII (Haemophilia A and B and von Willebrand's disease most common inherited coagulation defects)
- Circulating anticoagulant – lupus anticoagulant
- Oral anticoagulants (warfarin) – moderate prolongation of APTT
- Vitamin K deficiency

Common causes of a prolonged PT
- Oral anticoagulant drugs (warfarin) – Vitamin K antagonists
- Liver disease, especially obstructive
- Vitamin K deficiency
- DIC
- Factor VII, V, X or prothrombin defect
- Heparin will increase PT if in excess
- Massive blood transfusion

Primary Antiphospholipid Syndrome

Q 13. **Which of the following is not a feature of primary antiphospholipid syndrome?**

A. Pulmonary hypertension
B. Transient ischaemic attacks
C. Severe pre-eclampsia
D. Neutropenia
E. Thrombocytopenia

Q 14. **A young woman presents with a deep venous thrombosis. Which of the following factors is unlikely to have contributed to this?**

A. A recent holiday in Australia
B. Diabetes mellitus
C. The oral contraceptive pill
D. Paroxysmal nocturnal haemoglobinuria
E. A family history of venous thrombosis

A 13. **D**

Neutropenia is not a clinical feature of primary antiphospholipid syndrome, but can be a feature of rheumatoid arthritis in conjunction with splenomegaly as part of Felty's syndrome.

A 14. **B**

Diabetes mellitus is associated with arterial and not venous thromboses. A family history of thrombosis may imply the patient has an inherited thrombophilia. Paroxysmal nocturnal haemoglobinuria and the oral contraceptive pill are associated with venous thrombosis. Long haul flights have been associated with venous thromboses due to 'economy class syndrome'.

Primary antiphospholipid syndrome
- Diagnosis is based on presence of one clinical AND one serological criteria
- Clinical criteria are venous thrombosis, arterial thrombosis or recurrent miscarriage
- Venous thrombosis may be in unusual places eg Budd-Chiari, pulmonary hypertension due to multiple pulmonary emboli
- Stroke is the most prevalent result of arterial thrombosis, and transient ischaemic events may be a feature
- Pregnancy morbidity includes early and late miscarriages, intrauterine growth retardation and early severe pre-eclampsia
- Other clinical features include thrombocytopenia, livedo reticularis, migraine, chorea, epilepsy and endocardial disease, in particular valvular abnormalities
- Serological criteria are the presence of lupus anticoagulant or anticardiolipin IgG or IgM antibodies
- Lupus anticoagulant activity is detected via clotting based assays and ELISAs are used for the detection of anticardiolipin antibodies
- Both tests must be used as many cases of antiphospholipid antibody syndrome have either lupus anticoagulant or anticardiolipin antibody positivity and not both
- Venous or arterial thromboses should be treated with anticoagulation therapy. Pregnancy failure should be treated with aspirin and heparin

Causes of venous thrombosis
- Malignancy
- Pregnancy, obesity
- Trauma, surgery and immobility
- Paroxysmal nocturnal haemoglobinuria
- Deficiencies of antithrombin, protein C, protein S, plasminogen
- Activated protein C resistance (Factor V Leiden abnormality)
- Raised factor VIII levels
- Prothrombin polymorphism and dysfibrinogenaemia
- Drugs eg heparin induced thrombocytopenia

Causes of arterial or venous thrombosis
- Systemic lupus erythematosus/Antiphospholipid syndrome
- Behcets
- Homocysteinaemia
- Oestrogens (oral contraceptive pill)
- Polycythaemia
- Myelofibrosis
- Decreased fibrinolytic activity

Monoclonal Paraprotein

Q 15. A 74-year-old woman is referred to the haematology clinic after she was found to have a monoclonal paraprotein band. Which of the following conditions is least likely to be the underlying diagnosis?

- A. Systemic lupus erythematosus
- B. CMV infection
- C. Chronic myeloid leukaemia
- D. Non Hodgkin's lymphoma
- E. Gaucher's disease

Q 16. Which of the following statements about multiple myeloma is true:

- A. The incidence of multiple myeloma is higher in women than in men
- B. Hyperviscosity is most common in IgA myeloma
- C. Amyloidosis occurs in over 20% of patients with myeloma
- D. Bone scan is a useful investigation to stage disease
- E. Beta-2 microglobulin is a useful prognostic test

A 15. **C**

Monoclonal paraprotein bands are common in other lymphoproliferative conditions as well as myeloma and in 65% of cases are not associated with an underlying neoplastic disease. Chronic myeloid leukaemia is not associated with a monoclonal paraprotein band.

A 16. **E**

Multiple myeloma is more common in men than in women. Hyperviscosity is most common in IgM myeloma because of its pentameric structure. Amyloidosis occurs in less than 5% of patients with myeloma and is most common in those with IgA and Bence Jones Protein disease. Bone scan is not a useful investigation in myeloma and will not reveal lytic lesions. It is only useful to diagnose fractures which will show up as hot spots. A skeletal survey is the radiological investigation of choice in myeloma. A raised B2 microglobulin is one of the poor prognostic factors in myeloma.

Causes of paraproteinaemia

Lymphoproliferative disorders
- Myeloma
- Waldenstrom's macroglobulinaemia
- Chronic lymphatic leukaemia
- Lymphoma
- Heavy-chain disease
- Primary amyloidosis

Benign monoclonal gammopathies

Reactive
- Non lymphoid neoplasms eg carcinoma colon
- Infection eg Cytomegalovirus, tuberculosis
- Autoimmune disease eg systemic lupus erythematosus
- Liver disease eg hepatitis, cirrhosis
- Gaucher's disease

Idiopathic
- Monoclonal gammopathy of undetermined significance

Myeloma
- Median age of diagnosis is 70 years
- Diagnosis is made in the presence of two of monoclonal protein in blood or urine, 10% plasma cells in bone marrow and lytic bone lesions
- Other clinical features are bone disease, hypercalcaemia, renal failure, bone marrow failure and immune paresis
- 5 year survival is only 25%
- Treatment is supportive, chemotherapy (which can be oral or intravenous) and autologous or allogeneic stem cell transplantation
- Thalidomide has recently been used in relapsed and refractory disease

Leukaemias

Q 17. Which of the following features is **not** a characteristic of chronic myeloid leukaemia?

    A. There is a spectrum of myeloid cells in the peripheral blood, with a preponderance of mature cells

    B. NAP score is low

    C. Basophilia

    D. Chromosomal translocation t (9;21)

    E. Splenomegaly

Q 18. You are asked to discuss the possibility of using the drug, imatinib, with a patient and his family. Which of the following statements is most accurate?

    A. Imatinib is an inhibitor of tyrosine kinases and is used in the treatment of chronic lymphocytic leukaemia

    B. Imatinib is an inhibitor of tyrosine kinases associated with PML:RARa, and is used in the treatment of chronic myeloid leukaemia

    C. Imatinib is an inhibitor of tyrosine kinases associated with bcr-abl and is used in the treatment of chronic myeloid leukaemia

    D. Imatinib is a promotor of tyrosine kinases and is used in the treatment of chronic myeloid leukaemia

    E. Imatinib is a promotor of tyrosine kinases and is used in the treatment of acute lymphoblastic leukaemia

A 17. D

Chronic myeloid is characterized by a spectrum of myeloid cells in the peripheral blood, with a preponderance of mature cells and often a peak of neutrophils and of myelocytes. Small numbers of promyelocytes and blasts may be present. Splenomegaly is seen in 60–80% of patients on diagnosis and may be massive. Basophilia is common and NAP (neutrophil alkaline phosphatase) score, a cytochemical test is low. The characteristic chromosomal translocation is t (9;22).

A 18. C

Imatinib is an exciting new drug used in the treatment of chronic myeloid leukaemia (CML). It is an inhibitor of the tyrosine kinases associated with *Bcr-Abl* the genetic defect in CML. The *Bcr-Abl* kinase is thought to play a dominant role in the deregulated myeloid cell proliferation which is the hallmark of this disease. If there is inhibition of tyrosine kinase activity, there is control of myeloid cell proliferation. In clinical trials, over 50% of patients with chronic phase CML refractory to interferon attained a haematological remission with imatinib and many also achieved a cytogenetic response. Further clinical trials are now underway.

Chronic myeloid leukaemia
- 20% of all leukaemia
- Chromosomal abnormality is the translocation t(9;22) which is seen in over 90% of cases
- Philadelphia chromosome is the abnormal chromosome 22
- The underlying molecular defect is the BCR-ABL translocation
- Median age of onset is 40–50 years and 50% of patients are asymptomatic at diagnosis
- Clinical features include weight loss, lassitude, anorexia, night sweats, splenomegaly and features of anaemia, thrombocytopenia and hyperviscosity
- Features of hyperviscosity include visual disturbance, stroke or priapism
- Treatment includes hydroxyurea, interferon and imatinib
- Allogeneic stem cell transplantation is the only curative option
- Median survival from diagnosis is 5–6 years and patients progress from chronic phase to accelerated phase and blast crisis
- Death is due to terminal acute transformation to acute lymphoblastic or acute myeloid leukaemia or from bone marrow failure

Chronic Lymphocytic Leukaemia

Q 19. Which of the following statements about chronic lymphocytic leukaemia is true?

A. It has a peak incidence in patients of 40–50 years of age
B. The majority of patients are symptomatic at diagnosis with lymphadenopathy and night sweats
C. Auto immune haemolytic anaemia occurs in 10–15% of patients
D. About 50% of patients develop acute leukaemia as a terminal event
E. Median survival is 10–12 years

Q 20. A 77-year-old woman is referred to your clinic by her GP. A routine FBC showed a lymphocyte count of 56 × 10^9/l with 18% prolymphocytes and smear cells on blood film. Which of the following is not a poor prognostic factor?

A. Female sex
B. Age over 70 years
C. Lymphocyte count >50 × 10^9/l
D. Prolymphocytes comprising more than 10% of the peripheral blood lymphocytes
E. Lymphocyte doubling time less than 12 months

A 19. **C**

Chronic lymphocytic leukaemia is chiefly a disease of the elderly. Patients are often asymptomatic at diagnosis and in over 30% of patients it is an incidental finding. Auto immune haemolytic anaemia does occur in 10–15% of patients and has a positive Direct Coomb's test, spherocytes and a reticulocytosis. Median survival is 3–5 years and death is usually due to infection because of bone marrow failure and immune deficiency. Small numbers transform to more aggressive disease which is usually prolymphocytic leukaemia or large cell lymphoma, not acute leukaemia.

A 20. **A**

Male sex is a poor prognostic factor as are the other factors listed.

Chronic lymphocytic leukaemia
- Constitutes 25% of all leukaemias. It is chiefly a disease of the elderly
- It is characterised by an accumulation of mature lymphocytes in the peripheral blood, bone marrow, spleen, liver and lymph nodes
- Clinical findings include painless, symmetrical lymphadenopathy, hepatosplenomegaly, pruritus and symptoms due to bone marrow failure
- Blood film will show large numbers of mature lymphocytes and smear or smudge cells. Anaemia and thrombocytopenia are common
- Hypogammaglobulinaemia is common and monoclonal paraproteins are occasionally seen
- Staging is by the Binet or Rai systems and depends on number of areas involved and full blood count results
- Median survival is 3–5 years and one-third die of causes other than the leukaemia
- In early stages no treatment is required. In later stages and in rapidly progressive disease treatment is with oral or intravenous chemotherapy such as chlorambucil or fludarabine. Stem cell transplantation is an option in younger patients

Acute Myeloid Leukaemia

Q 21. Which of the following statements about acute myeloid leukaemia is true?

A. The peripheral blood film in acute myeloid leukaemia is characterised by spectrum of myeloid cells with a preponderance of mature myeloid cells
B. Auer rods are pathognomonic of acute myeloid leukaemia
C. 80% of childhood leukaemia is acute myeloid leukaemia
D. Remission rates of about 50% are achieved for patients under the age of 60 years
E. Central nervous system disease is very common and patients must be given prophylactic therapy

Q 22. A 45-year-old lady is admitted to hospital with a DIC-like coagulopathy. Fibrinogen levels are low with normal AT III and protein C levels. Film shows circulating myeloblasts with Auer rods. A diagnosis of acute promyelocytic leukaemia is made. Which of the following statements is true? Acute promyelocytic leukaemia:

A. is a subtype of acute myeloid leukaemia with a poor prognosis
B. usually presents with a very high white cell count
C. is associated with a particular cytogenetic translocation involving chromosomes 9 and 22
D. is associated with a fusion of the PMC and RARα genes
E. is best treated with combination chemotherapy

A 21. B

Auer rods are indeed pathognomonic of acute myeloid leukaemia. The peripheral blood described is characteristic of chronic myeloid leukaemia. 80% of adult acute leukaemia is myeloid, but 80% of childhood leukaemia is acute lymphoblastic leukaemia. Remission rates of 80–85% are achieved for patients under the age of 60 years. Central nervous system disease is very common in acute lymphoblastic leukaemia and these patients receive prophylactic therapy.

A 22. D

Acute promyelocytic leukaemia is subtype M3 of acute myeloid leukaemia. It is associated with the chromosomal translocation t(15;17). It used to have a poor prognosis because of the presence of prominent disseminated coagulation at diagnosis, but with aggressive treatment of the coagulopathy and treatment with all-trans retinoic acid (ATRA) in addition to standard chemotherapy, it now carries a good prognosis.

Acute myeloid leukaemia
- Presentation is often with clinical features of bone marrow failure and anaemia and thrombocytopenia are often profound
- Myeloblasts are usually present in the peripheral blood, but the patient may present with an aplastic picture
- Diagnosis is based on the presence of more than 20% myeloblasts in the bone marrow aspirate
- Classification is based on morphological, immunological and cytogenetic criteria and it is subdivided into 8 categories, M0 to M7
- Treatment tends to be more intensive than for acute lymphoblastic leukaemia and to achieve a complete remission a profound (if transient) bone marrow hypoplasia must be obtained
- Combinations of chemotherapeutic drugs are given in 4 or 5 successive courses. Following each course of treatment the patient is severely neutropenic for 1–2 weeks and needs hospital admission and protective isolation
- New approaches to treatment include drug modifying agents and monoclonal antibody therapy

Acute promyelocytic leukaemia
- M3 variant of acute myeloid leukaemia
- Mean age of presentation is 25 years (younger than other types of acute myeloid leukaemia)
- It tends to present with pancytopenia and a low white count in the peripheral blood, but there are large numbers of promyelocytes in the bone marrow, which are heavily granulated with prominent Auer rods
- Disseminated intravascular coagulation is seen in 80% at diagnosis with severe haemorrhagic manifestations

It is associated with a translocation of chromosomes 15 and 17, and the molecular defect is a fusion of the PML and RARα genes.

Acute Lymphoblastic Leukaemia

Q 23. Which of these is not a common presenting symptom of acute lymphoblastic leukaemia?

    A. Bone and joint pain
    B. Lymphadenopathy
    C. Mediastinal masses
    D. Gum hypertrophy
    E. Testicular swelling

Q 24. Which of these is a poor prognostic factor in acute lymphoblastic leukaemia?

    A. The presence of the Philadelphia chromosomal translocation t(9;22)
    B. Female sex
    C. Age between 3 and 5 years
    D. Pancytopenia at presentation
    E. Common ALL subtype

A 23. **D**

Gum hypertrophy is more frequently in the monocytic subtypes of acute myeloid leukaemia, M4 (acute myelomonocytic leukaemia) and M5 (acute monocytic/monoblastic leukaemia). The other symptoms are common presenting features of acute lymphoblastic leukaemia. Bone pain is seen in about 50% of patients at presentation and the presence of joint pain often leads to initial investigation for rheumatoid arthritis. Lymphadenopathy is seen in 65% of patients and mediastinal masses are seen in patients with T-cell disease. Testicular swelling is common as the testes are sanctuary sites for the leukaemic cells.

A 24. **A**

The presence of the Philadelphia chromosome is a poor prognostic factor in acute lymphoblastic leukaemia. Other poor prognostic factors are male sex, age less than 1 year or over 50 years, meningeal involvement at diagnosis, T-ALL subtype, initial high white count and failure to respond rapidly to treatment. NOTE: The Philadelphia Chromosome is more commonly associated with C.M.L. where it is not a poor prognostic factor.

Acute lymphoblastic leukaemia
- This is the commonest type of leukaemia in children with a peak incidence at 4–5 years of age
- A higher incidence of acute lymphoblastic and acute myeloid leukaemia are seen in children with Down's syndrome
- Clinical features may be due to bone marrow infiltration (infections, anaemia and haemorrhagic symptoms) or due to organ infiltration (bone pain, joint pain, lymphadenopathy, hepatosplenomegaly, meningeal syndrome, testicular swelling and mediastinal masses)
- The white blood count is usually raised at presentation with large numbers of primitive cells (lymphoid blasts), although the patient may be pancytopenic. The bone marrow is hypercellular with large numbers of blasts. Lytic bone lesions may be seen on X-rays
- Immunological and cytogenetic markers are crucial for subclassification and are important for prognosis. Acute lymphoblastic is divided into B and T cell lineage
- Treatment is initially with supportive care (antibiotics, blood products) and with chemotherapeutic regimens. These comprise of remission induction therapy which is usually achieved without myelotoxicity in the majority of cases. This is followed with consolidation with more intensive chemotherapy, maintenance therapy (which is continued for 2 years) and central nervous system directed therapy. The latter treatment may be cranial irradiation or intravenous and intrathecal methotrexate
- Disease free survival is achieved in between 55 and 75% of children, but prognosis is much worse in adults

Non-Hodgkin's Lymphoma

Q 25. All of the following infections are associated with Non-Hodgkin's lymphoma except:

A. Brucellosis
B. *Helicobacter pylori*
C. Epstein-Barr virus
D. Human immunodeficiency virus
E. Human T-cell leukaemia virus

Q 26. Which of the following statements about Non-Hodgkin's lymphoma is true?

A. Non-Hodgkin's lymphoma has the highest incidence between 10 and 30 years
B. The finding of a raised lactate dehydrogenase level is common in non-Hodgkin's lymphoma
C. A monoclonal paraprotein is found in over 40% of cases of non-Hodgkin's lymphoma
D. One treatment option in non-Hodgkin's lymphoma is the use of a monoclonal antibody against CD33
E. The lymphadenopathy in non-Hodgkin's lymphoma is usually asymmetrical and painful

A 25. **A**

Brucellosis may be associated with lymphadenopathy but does not cause lymphoma. *Helicobacter pylori* can cause gastric lymphoma due to chronic antigenic stimulation resulting from persistent bacterial infection. Epstein-Barr virus is associated with Burkitt's lymphoma and lymphoma in the immunosuppressed. HIV infection is associated with an increased risk of lymphoma. HTLV infection is associated with adult T-cell leukaemia/lymphoma.

A 26. **B**

The incidence of non-Hodgkin's lymphoma rises with increased age. This condition is associated with widespread painless lymphadenopathy, a raised lactate dehydrogenase level and a paraprotein in between 5 and 15% of cases. One treatment option is the use of rituximab, a monoclonal antibody aimed against CD20.

Non-Hodgkin's lymphoma
- There has been a dramatic increase in incidence of this condition since the 1970s partially due to HIV infection. It may occur at any age but incidence rises considerably with age
- Median age of presentation is 55–60 years and it classically presents with widespread painless lymphadenopathy and hepatosplenomegaly
- B symptoms are unexplained fever of 38° or higher, night sweats sufficient to waken the patient from sleep and loss of more than 10% of body weight in the 6 months prior to diagnosis
- Investigations may reveal circulating lymphoma cells, pancytopenia, an autoimmune haemolytic anaemia, hypoalbuminaemia, raised LDH and a paraprotein
- Staging is based on the Ann Arbor staging system for Hodgkin's disease and is stage I to IV dependent on extent of disease and A or B depending on symptom status
- Classification is complicated but based on the REAL classification of 1994 (updated in the WHO classification of 2000). Non-Hodgkin's lymphoma is divided into B and T cell neoplasms and each of these is subdivided into several types
- Management depends on stage and nature of the lymphoma. Indolent disease is treated only if advanced and symptomatic. Treatment options include oral therapy with chlorambucil, fludarabine or cyclophosphamide or with combination intravenous therapies. In addition monoclonal antibody therapy (rituximab – anti CD20) and stem cell transplantation may be used
- In histologically aggressive disease combination chemotherapy is usually used. Stem cell transplantation is of use in patients with relapsed or resistant disease

Hodgkin's Lymphoma/Blood Transfusion

Q 27. Which of the following statements about Hodgkin's lymphoma is true?

    A. The incidence of Hodgkin's lymphoma increases with increased age

    B. Eosinophilia is commonly seen in Hodgkin's lymphoma

    C. The presence of pruritus is a poor prognostic factor in Hodgkin's lymphoma

    D. The presence of alcohol induced lymph node pain is a poor prognostic factor in Hodgkin's lymphoma

    E. Hodgkin's lymphoma can only be diagnosed if Reed-Sternberg cells are seen in the lymph node biopsy

Q 28. Which of the following infections are currently routinely tested for in donated blood?

    A. Malaria

    B. Syphilis

    C. Hepatitis A

    D. Parvovirus

    E. HTLV I and II

A 27. **B**

In the UK the incidence of Hodgkin's disease rises in adolescence and peaks in the third decade. In developing countries the peak incidence is in childhood. Eosinophilia is commonly seen in Hodgkin's disease. Pruritus and alcohol induced lymph node pain are common symptoms in Hodgkin's disease, but are of no prognostic significance and are not B symptoms. Although Reed-Sternberg cells are pathognomic of Hodgkin's disease, it can be diagnosed in their absence if other characteristic features are present.

A 28. **B**

In the UK the infectious agents that are currently routinely tested for are treponema pallidum (syphilis), Hepatitis B and C, HIV and CMV. CMV is important in the immunosuppressed patient, so these patients are issued CMV negative blood. Malaria parasites are easily transmitted by blood transfusion and currently donors are carefully vetted with direct questioning. Donors who have lived in endemic areas or who have had an attack of malaria can be accepted and their plasma used, but the red cells must not be issued. Visitors who have recently travelled to a tropical area are treated similarly for 12 months after their return. Hepatitis A is rarely transmitted by transfusion. Any donor who has been in close contact with a case or develops hepatitis A is deferred for 12 months. Parvovirus can be transmitted by blood transfusion but is only a clinical issue in patients with shortened red cell survival. In areas of low prevalence of HTLV infection the value of screening is not clear and this test is not currently mandatory in the UK.

Hodgkin's lymphoma
- Hodgkin's lymphoma presents most commonly with supradiaphragmatic lymph node involvement and lymph nodes are classically firm, rubbery and often bulky
- B symptoms are as with non-Hodgkin's lymphoma and correlate with stage, disease bulk and prognosis
- Full blood count may reveal anaemia, lymphopenia and eosinophilia. The ESR is commonly raised and the LDH may be raised. The bone marrow is usually normal
- Staging is done using the Ann Arbor system, stages I to IV and symptom status A or B
- Classification of Hodgkin's lymphoma is done with the REAL classification into 5 subtypes
- Early stage disease is treated with radiotherapy or a combination of radiotherapy and chemotherapy. Advanced disease is treated with combination chemotherapy and stem cell transplantation in relapsed or refractory disease

Myelodysplasia/Polycythaemia

Q 29. A 65-year-old male patient is diagnosed as having myelodysplasia. Which of the following statements about this condition is true?

A. Myelodysplasia has its highest incidence in patients of 40–50 years of age
B. The majority of patients with myelodysplasia present with isolated thrombocytopenia
C. Myelodysplasia is a pre-leukaemic condition
D. The median survival in myelodysplasia is 5–6 years
E. The majority of patients with myelodysplasia die from unrelated causes

Q 30. Which of the following patients is most likely to have polycythaemia rubra vera?

A. 55 year old man with a packed cell volume of 0.55%, a raised red cell mass, a history of chronic renal failure and a raised level of erythropoietin
B. 55 year old man with a packed cell volume of 0.55%, a raised red cell mass, a platelet count of $600 \times 10^9/l$ and splenomegaly
C. 55 year old woman with a packed cell volume of 0.53%, a raised red cell mass and a history of fibroids
D. 55 year old man with a packed cell volume of 0.55%, a normal red cell mass and a history of hypertension
E. 25 year old man with a packed cell volume of 0.57%, a raised red cell mass and a history of congenital heart disease

[A] 29. **C**

Myelodysplasia is a pre-leukaemic condition and has an increased incidence with increasing age. The majority of patients present with features of bone marrow failure and isolated thrombocytopenia is a presenting feature in less than 5% of patients. The median survival in myelodysplasia is 20 months and the majority of patients die from complication of bone marrow failure.

[A] 30. **B**

Polycythaemia rubra vera is a myeloproliferative disorder diagnosed in patients with a raised packed cell volume, raised red cell mass and normal plasma volume. It is often associated with a thrombocytosis and splenomegaly. It must be differentiated from apparent polycythaemia where the red cell mass is within the normal range, but packed cell volume is high because of a reduced plasma volume. This is often seen in patients with a history of smoking, high alcohol intake and hypertension (Case D). Secondary polycythaemia is characterised by a raised red cell mass but this is secondary to a raised erythropoietin level. This may be due to appropriate secretion of erythropoietin as in cyanotic congenital heart disease (Case E), hypoxic lung disease and at high altitude. It may also be due to inappropriate secretion of erthropoietin from renal tumours and in renal ischaemia (Case A), hepatomas, fibroids (Case C), bronchial carcinomas and phaeochromocytomas.

Myelodysplasia
- This pre-leukaemic condition is due to a disorder of the multipotent haemopoietic stem cell
- 20% of patients with myelodysplasia are diagnosed from an incidental blood count but the majority of patients present with features of bone marrow failure. Anaemia is very common and is often macrocytic. Autoimmune features can be a problem. Peripheral blood shows abnormal appearances of blood cells in all lineages
- The WHO classification (2000) uses the presence of blasts in peripheral blood and bone marrow and the presence of ring sideroblasts in the bone marrow to form subtypes of myelodysplasia. This is important for prognosis
- Median survival in myelodysplasia is 20 months. 70–80% of patients die of marrow failure and about 30% transform to acute leukaemia
- Treatment is often supportive with transfusion therapy and antibiotics if required. In younger patients cytotoxic chemotherapy or stem cell transplantation are used

Polycythaemia rubra vera:
- Splenomegaly
- Aquagenic pruritus
- Bleeding
- Gout
- Peptic ulcer
- Conversion to myelofibrosis or leukaemia in 10%

Infectious Diseases

Microbiology and Infectious Diseases

Soft Tissue Infection

Q 1. A 50-year-old man with NIDDM develops severe pain and erythema around a recent laporotomy wound, a plain X-ray shows gas in the soft tissues. Which is the least likely diagnosis?

A. Fournier's gangrene
B. Necrotising fasciitis type I
C. Necrotising fasciitis type II
D. Clostridial gas gangrene
E. Surgical emphysema

Q 2. Which of the following is not a Group A streptococcal virulence factor?

A. Streptokinase
B. Hyaluronidase
C. M protein
D. Coagulase
E. SpeA

A 1. **C**

Necrotising fasciitis is a painful deep soft tissue infection characterised by destruction of fascia and fat. Necrotising fasciitis type I is a mixed infection due to aerobic and anaerobic bacteria occurring after surgery, especially in diabetics. Necrotising fasciitis type II is caused by Group A streptococci (*S. pyogenes*). It can occur in any age group and in the previously healthy. Gas in the soft tissues occurs in infections with a large anaerobic component, non-infectious causes include surgical emphysema, pneumothorax, pneumomediastinum, fractured larynx and fractured trachea.

A 2. **D**

Coagulase is a prothrombotic enzyme produced by *S. aureus,* also used in its laboratory identification. Streptokinase, produced by group A, C and G streptococci, converts plasminogen to plasmin which has fibrinolytic activity and activates the alternative complement pathway. *S. pyogenes* produces several pyrogenic exotoxins (SpeA, C, and F) implicated in streptococcal toxic shock syndrome. M proteins are found on the surface of Group A streptococci and may act as superantigens. An association between M phenotype and the development of post streptococcal syndromes (rheumatic fever and glomerulonephritis) has been observed.

A classification of soft tissue infections
Superficial
- Impetigo (*S. pyogenes, S. aureus*)
- Bullous impetigo (*S. aureus* phage group II)
- Folliculitis (*S. aureus, P. aeruginosa*)

Subcutaneous
- Abscesses/boils (*S. aureus*)
- Cellulitis (*S. aureus, S. pyogenes*)
- Erysipelas (*S. pyogenes* rarely group B, C or D Streps)
- Animal bites (*Pasteurella multocida, Capnocytophaga canimorsus*)
- Water exposure (*Aeromonas hydrophilla, Mycobacterium marinum*)
- Fish mongering (*Erysipelothrix rhusiopathiae*)

Deep
- Necrotising fasciitis type I (mixed anaerobes and aerobes)
- Necrotising fasciitis type II (*S. pyogenes*)
- Clostridial gas gangrene (*C. perfringens, C. septicum, C. novyi*)
- Fournier's gangrene (Coliforms, enterococci, *B. fragilis,* peptostreptococci)
- Meleney's synergistic gangrene (*S. aureus* and microaerophilic streptococci)
- Lemierre's syndrome – *Fusobacterium necrophorum* infection in the head and neck
- Pyomyositis – Occurs in tropical areas, usually due to *S. aureus*

Virulence factors in *S. pyogenes* and *S. aureus*

	S. pyogenes	*S. aureus*
Toxins	Pyrogenic exotoxins (SpeA, B, C, F) Streptolysin O	Cytotoxin Leukocidin Enterotoxins A-E Epidermolytic toxin
Enzymes	Streptokinase C5 peptidase	Coagulase Staphylokinase Hyaluronidase DNAase
Others	Cell wall – lipoteichoic acid M proteins	Cell wall – lipoteichoic acid Capsule Slime

Tuberculosis

Q 3. The following CSF results are obtained from a 55-year-old alcoholic. White cell count 240 × 10⁶/ml (75% lymphocytes), protein 5.6 g/l, glucose 2.6 mmol/l. Blood glucose 5.4 mmol/l. Gram stain, Ziehl-Nielson stain, cryptococcal antigen and culture are negative. What is the most appropriate investigation?

- **A.** Auramine staining of induced sputum
- **B.** Mantoux test
- **C.** TB PCR on CSF
- **D.** Bone marrow aspiration and culture
- **E.** Early morning urine culture

Q 4. A patient with suspected tuberculosis underwent a Mantoux test. A negative result could result from all the following except:

- **A.** Sarcoidosis
- **B.** Hodgkin's disease
- **C.** Prior immunisation with BCG
- **D.** Miliary tuberculosis
- **E.** Hypoalbuminaemia

A 3. **C**

A moderate CSF lymphocytosis, high protein and low glucose are seen in TB meningitis (TBM). Direct ZN staining of CSF is insensitive and positive in only 10–20% of culture proven cases. Culture is the gold standard but too slow (6–8 weeks) to delay initiation of therapy. Rapid diagnosis is best achieved by PCR which has a sensitivity of 75% and a specificity of 94%. Skin tests are usually negative in TBM. TBM occurs due to reactivation of old disease or accompanying miliary tuberculosis in which case mycobacteria may be isolated from other sites, e.g. bone marrow, urine or sputum.

A 4. **C**

Prior administration of BCG may lead to a false positive Mantoux test. The degree of positivity wanes with time so vaccinated individuals with strongly positive skin tests should be investigated for other evidence of tuberculosis, e.g. CXR, especially if they were vaccinated in infancy.

Causes of a false-negative Mantoux test
Non-specific
- Age >70 years or <1 year
- Hypoalbuminaemia <2 g/dl
- Anaemia
- Fever
- Chronic renal failure
- Leukocytosis >15,000

Infections
- HIV, rubella, EBV, mumps, VZV, influenza
- Miliary TB
- Disseminated mycoses

Other diseases
- Malignancies – Hodgkin's, leukaemia
- Sarcoidosis

Drugs
- Immunosuppressives – corticosteroids
- Recent live viral vaccination – MMR, oral polio
- Radiotherapy

Testing errors
- Poor injection technique
- Error in measuring skin induration
- Test performed too early in infection (<10 weeks)
- Out of date tuberculin

Hepatitis B

Q 5. A surgeon has the following hepatitis B serology. HBsAg +ve, Anti-HBs +ve, Anti-HBc +ve, HBeAg −ve, Anti-HBe +ve. Which of the following statements is correct?

A. The surgeon may perform exposure prone procedures
B. He is immune due to hepatitis B vaccination
C. Household contacts should be given hepatitis B vaccine and hepatitis B immunoglobulin
D. A viral load test should be performed
E. He has acute hepatitis B infection

Q 6. Which of the following statements about hepatitis B is true?

A. Liver biopsy is indicated in all carriers with abnormal liver enzymes
B. There is a strong association with porphyria cutanea tarda
C. 40% of individuals infected in adulthood develop chronic disease
D. Viral replication does not involve a reverse transcriptase
E. Therapy with interferon-alpha is most effective in carriers with little inflammation on liver biopsy

A 5. **D**

He has been naturally infected with hepatitis B (anti-HBc +ve) and has remained a carrier (HBsAg +ve). He has a low risk of infectivity as he is HBeAg −ve, household contacts should be screened and given hepatitis B vaccine alone, sexual contacts should receive vaccine and hepatitis B immunoglobulin. Healthcare workers with pre-core mutant viruses, which do not produce HBeAg, have been associated with transmission to patients, under new health service guidelines they cannot undertake exposure prone procedures unless their HBV DNA is less than 10^3 copies/ml.

A 6. **A**

Only a small percentage (5–10%) become carriers if infected in adulthood, compared with 90% of those infected perinatally. Liver biopsy to detect cirrhosis or hepatocellular carcinoma is indicated in all carriers with abnormal LFT's, liver ultrasound or detectable HBV DNA. Immune complex deposition may lead to vasculitis, polyarthritis nodosum and glomerulonephritis. Porphyria cutanea tarda and lichen planus are associated with hepatitis C infection. The virus has a complicated lifecycle; HBV DNA is not transcribed directly, it is converted to +ve sense ssRNA and then by a viral reverse transcriptase to dsDNA which can be directly transcribed by the host cell.

Hepatitis B virus
- Double stranded DNA virus
- Spread by sexual intercourse, blood and IVDU. Highest incidence SE Asia and Africa due to vertical transmission
- Incubation period 40 to 160 days
- Insidious onset, jaundice in 25% of adults
- Extra hepatic complications – polyarteritis nodosa, polyarthralgia, glomerulonephritis due to immune complex deposition
- 1% develop fulminant hepatitis, 5–10% become carriers
- HBV carriers should be monitored for evidence of viral replication with yearly serology (HBeAg), HBV DNA and LFT's
- Abnormal LFT's are an indication for liver biopsy to assess degree of inflammation
- Interferon-alpha is effective in reducing viral replication in 20–40% of patients. Response is better in females v males, <50 years age, Low HBV DNA levels and a high degree of inflammation on liver biopsy

Hepatitis B serology
- 3 antigens associated with the surface (HBsAg), and core (HBcAg and HBeAg) of the virus
- Presence of HBeAg is strongly associated with high infectivity and progression to chronic liver disease

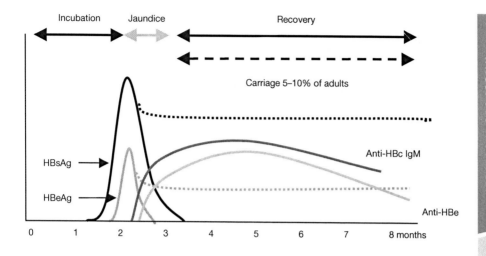

Interpretation of Hepatitis B serology

	HBsAg	Anti-HBs	Anti-HBc	Anti-HBc IgM	HBeAg	Anti-HBe
Incubation	+	−	−	−	+	−
Acute infection	+	−	+	+++	+	−
Natural recovery	−	+	+	−	−	−
Carrier low infectivity	+	−	+	−	−	+/−
Carrier high infectivity	+	−	+	−	+	+/−
Immunised	−	+	−	−	−−	−

Fever and Lymphadenopathy

Q 7. 2 weeks after returning from a trip to North Africa a 23-year-old
student presents with flu like symptoms, myalgia and posterior
cervical lymphadenopathy. Temperature 38.4°C, Hb 14.0 g/dl,
White cell count 8.5 × 10⁹/l platelets 150 × 10⁹/l, ESR 5 mm/h,
CRP <5 mg/l. What is the most likely diagnosis?

A. Brucellosis
B. Toxoplasmosis
C. Typhoid fever
D. Epstein Barr virus infection
E. Leptospirosis

Q 8. Which statement is true regarding fever of unknown origin?

A. It is defined as temperature >37.5°C on 3 consecutive days
    with no identifiable focus of infection
B. An infection is the cause in 70% of cases
C. Eosinophilia is diagnostic of a parasitic infection
D. Patients should be started on broad spectrum antibiotics
E. A relapsing fever is suggestive of lymphoma

A 7. B

Acute toxoplasmosis may present as a mononucleosis-like syndrome with lethargy, fever and headache. The lymphadenopathy is characteristically posterior cervical. White cell count, CRP and ESR are usually normal, a raised white cell count (lymphocytosis) would be expected in EBV infection. Systemic bacterial diseases, e.g. brucellosis, typhoid and leptospirosis may present with similar symptoms accompanied by generalised lymphadenopathy and raised inflammatory markers.

A 8. E

Only a few conditions are associated with a distinct fever pattern. Recurrent fever over days or weeks occurs with lymphoma (Pel-Ebstein fever), tertian or quartan malaria and brucellosis. A biphasic fever occurs in dengue and leptospirosis. Although eosinophilia suggests a parasitic infection it may also occur in drug fevers and lymphoma. Only about 30% of FUO's have an infectious origin, and there is no rational for the routine administration of antibiotics. Resolution of fever may be wrongly ascribed to antibiotic administration, delay diagnosis and lead to a false sense of security. There is no uniform set of investigations in the patient with FUO; the most successful approach is observation and repeated clinical examination for new diagnostic clues.

Causes of lymphadenopathy
- Bacterial infections – localised pyogenic infection, secondary syphilis, tuberculosis, bartonellosis, chancroid, plague, tularaemia
- Viral infections – EBV, CMV, HIV, pharyngoconjunctival fever (adenovirus), rubella, genital herpes (HSV-2), HHV-6
- Other infections – lymphogranuloma venereum, spotted fever, histoplasmosis, coccidiodomycosis, toxoplasmosis, leishmaniasis, Chagas disease, filariasis, onchocerciacis
- Malignancies – lymphoma, leukaemia, metastatic disease
- Others – sarcoidosis, SLE, Kawasaki's disease, Castleman's disease, drug allergy, amyloidosis, dermatomyositis, hyperthyroidism, Addison's disease

Fever of unknown origin
- Beeson and Petersdorf criteria – T >38.3°C for at least 3 weeks and failure to establish a diagnosis after 1 week of investigation

Causes
- Infections 30% – focal bacterial infection (cholangitis, prostatitis), tuberculosis, endocarditis, abdominal abscesses, HIV, PCP, atypical mycobacteria, typhoid, amoebiasis, disseminated candidiasis, toxoplasmosis, EBV, CMV, Lyme disease
- Malignancy 20% – Hodgkin's and NHL, renal cell carcinoma, colonic carcinoma, atrial myxoma, leiomyosarcoma

- Collagen disorders 10% – adult stills, RA, relapsing polychondritis, temporal arteritis, Wegener's granulomatosis, polyarteritis nodosa, SLE, polymyalgia rheumatica
- Others 20% – granulomatous diseases (Crohn's, sarcoidosis, granulomatous hepatitis), subacute thyroiditis, pulmonary embolus, Familial Mediterranean fever, retroperitoneal haematoma, drugs (antibiotics, phenytoin, atropine, procainamide), factitious fever, hyperthyroidism, cyclical neutropenia
- Undiagnosed 30% – most will resolve spontaneously

Respiratory Infection

Q 9. **Which of the following statement is false?**

A. *Mycoplasma pneumoniae* infection is associated with bullous myringitis
B. *Burkholderia cepacia* infects patients with cystic fibrosis
C. *Legionella pneumophila* infection is more common in smokers
D. *Chlamydia pneumoniae* infection is associated with exposure to birds
E. *Acinetobacter baumaniae* causes outbreaks of nosocomial pneumonia

Q 10. **As the medical registrar on call you are referred a 40 yr old man from A&E with a diagnosis of community acquired pneumonia. Which of the following parameters is not associated with a poor outcome?**

A. Multi-lobar involvement on chest X-ray
B. Bacteraemia
C. Blood urea 13 mmol/l
D. Blood pressure 90/60 mmHg
E. White blood cell count 25 × 10⁹/l

A 9. D

Psittacosis due to *Chlamydia psittaci* is associated with exposure to birds. *Chlamydia pneumonia* is a cause of atypical pneumonia in young adults and presents with cough, sore throat and bronchitis. *Mycoplasma pneumoniae* infection is associated with myringitis, encephalitis, ataxia and is a cause of erythema nodosum and erythema multiforme. *Burkholderia cepacia* may colonise the lungs of older cystic patients and is associated with rapid deterioration in lung function. It is highly transmissible and resistant to most antibiotics, requiring colonised patients to be treated in isolation and segregated clinics. *Acinetobacter baumanii* has been the cause of numerous outbreaks of nosocomial and ventilator associated pneumonia in intensive care units.

A 10. E

A white cell count of <4 or >30 × 10^9/l is associated with a poor outcome. Other factors include male sex, age >50 years, pre-existing medical disease, systolic hypotension or diastolic blood pressure <60 mmHg, PaO_2 <8 kPa, urea >7 mmol/l, bacteraemia, respiratory rate >30/min and multilobar involvement.

Community acquired pneumonia (CAP)
- *S. pneumoniae* is commonest cause of lobar pneumonia especially in healthy young adults
- Risk factors include ↑age, recent URTI (*S. aureus, H. influenzae*), COPD (*H. influenzae, M. catarrhalis*), alcoholism (*K. pneumoniae*) and cystic fibrosis (*S. aureus, P. aeruginosa*)
- 'Atypical pneumonia' refers to pneumonia unresponsive to penicillin without a bacteriological diagnosis. Causes include *Mycoplasma pneumoniae, Legionella pneumophila, Chlamydia pneumoniae, Chlamydia psittaci, Coxiella burnetti*, viruses
- Pneumococcal pneumonia presents with fever, cough and pleuritic chest pain or as an acute confusional state in the elderly. Consolidation and bronchial breathing may be found on examination and 50% develop pleural effusion
- Sore throat, headache and diarrhoea may be prominent symptoms of 'Atypical pneumonia', chest examination and CXR may be normal
- Cavitation on CXR suggests *S. aureus, K. pneumonia, M. tuberculosis,* lung abscess or a cavitating neoplasm
- Assessment of severity is based on respiratory rate, blood pressure, urea and electrolytes, blood gases and white cell count
- Current UK (BTS 2001) guidelines for antibiotic management
  - Non-severe pneumonia; oral amoxicillin + erythromycin
  - Severe pneumonia; IV co-amoxiclav or cefuroxime + erythromycin
  - β-lactam or macrolide intolerant; levofloaxacin
- Treat non-severe pneumonia for 7 days, severe for 10 and legionella, staphylococcal or Gram negative pneumonia for 14–21 days
- If the patient fails to improve repeat the CXR consider 1. alternative diagnosis, e.g. PE, pulmonary oedema, bronchial ca, bronchiectasis, 2. impaired immunity, e.g. HIV, myeloma, 3. complications, e.g. empyaema, lung abscess, ARDS, metastatic infection

Malaria

Q 11. A 28 yr old women returns from a trip to rural Thailand. She is admitted with fever and suspected malaria. Which of the following is true regarding *Plasmodium falciparum* infection?

A. Paroxysms of fever occur typically every 3rd day
B. Examination of multiple thin blood films is the most sensitive diagnostic test
C. Thrombocytopenia is rare in the absence of DIC
D. Corticosteroids should be administered in cerebral malaria
E. A parasitaemia of 5% warrants intravenous quinine therapy

Q 12. Regarding malaria which of the following is true?

A. *P. malariae* infection is treated with chloroquine followed by primaquine
B. After quinine treatment of *P. falciparum* infection pyrimethamine/sulfadoxine (Fansidar) is given to prevent relapse
C. Mefloquine resistance in *P. falciparum* is rare in South East Asia
D. Artemether may be given by the oral or intravenous route
E. Polymorphisms in the promoter region of the human tumour necrosis factor gene are associated with susceptibility to severe malaria

A 11. E

Fever occurring every 3rd day (benign tertian malaria) is a characteristic of *P. vivax* and *P. ovale* infection. Thick blood films are the most sensitive method of detecting malarial parasites, thin blood films are used to determine the species. Thrombocytopenia is very common in falciparum malaria without associated coagulation abnormalities. A parasitaemia of 5% is an indication of severe malaria and requires parenteral quinine therapy.

A 12. E

Relapse occurs in vivax and ovale infections due to reactivation of hypnozoites dormant in the liver. This is prevented by giving primaquine. Hypnozoites do not develop in falciparum infection but resurgence of malaria, known as recrudescence, due to asexual parasites resistant to quinine may occur. Pyrimethamine/sulfadoxine or doxycycline is given to prevent this. Individuals with a single nucleotide polymorphism in the TNF-α promoter are at increased risk of severe malaria. TNF-α stimulates the production of pro-inflammatory cytokines especially ICAM-1, which facilitate *P. falciparum* cytoadherence. High levels of TNF-α are associated with a poor outcome in falciparum malaria. High levels of resistance to all antimalarials including mefloquine are found in SE Asia. Artemisinin, under specialist guidance, may be used for severe drug resistant malaria in a returning traveller from this area of the world.

Malaria
- Life cycle: female Anopheles mosquito injects sporozoites which develop into exoerythrocytic hepatic schizonts in the liver. These release merozoites which invade red blood cells and form ring trophozoites and erythrocytic shizonts. Some merozoites develop into gametocytes which reproduce sexually when taken up by biting mosquitoes. *P. vivax* and *P. ovale* are able to lie dormant in the liver as hypnozoites
- Presents with paroxysmal fever, rigors, tachycardia and splenomegaly
- Complications of *P. falciparum*; cerebral malaria, hypoglycaemia, thrombocytopenia, pulmonary oedema, renal failure, Gram negative sepsis (algid malaria)
- Repeated thick and thin blood films needed for diagnosis and speciation. Other methods, able to detect plasmodium antigens in blood, include the parasite F and optimal tests

Antimalarials
- Chloroquine – used with primaquine for treatment of benign malarias and as prophylaxis in sensitive areas
- Quinine – treatment of choice for most falciparum malaria. Given with pyrimethamine/sulfadoxine for malaria form West Africa, or doxycycline for malaria from elsewhere, to prevent recrudescence

- Mefloquine – treatment of severe malaria with multidrug resistance and prophylaxis in chloroquine resistant areas
- Artemisinin – treatment of severe resistant malaria (in the UK only under exceptional circumstances). Can be given orally or by suppository. Artesunate is an IV preparation and artemether an IM form

Faecal Parasites

Q 13. An ultrasound scan shows dilated common bile ducts and a filling defect in the right lobe of the liver. Infection with which organism is unlikely to be associated with this lesion?

A. *Ascaris lumbricoides*
B. *Ankylostoma duodenale*
C. *Clonorchis sinensis*
D. *Entamoeba histolytica*
E. *Echinococcus granulosa*

Q 14. Which of the following statements is true?

A. *Strongyloides stercoralis* may present with Gram negative sepsis
B. Ingestion of undercooked pork infected with *Taenia soleum* leads directly to cysticercosis
C. *Entamoeba coli* may cause diarrhoea
D. *Cryptosporidium parvum* infection can be effectively treated with co-trimoxazole
E. *Diphyllobothrium latum* infection is associated with iron deficiency anaemia

A 13. **B**

Heavy infections with roundworm (*Ascaris lumbricoides*) and liver flukes (*Clonorchis sinensis, Fasciola hepatica*) can result in obstruction of the hepatic, pancreatic or common bile ducts and secondary abscess formation. *Entamoeba histolytica* forms amoebic liver abscesses and *Echinococcus granulosus* hydatid cysts most commonly in the liver. *Ankylostoma duodenale* (hookworm) infection may result in iron deficiency anaemia and hypoalbuminaemia in heavily infected or malnourished individuals.

A 14. **A**

The Strongyloides hyper-infection syndrome, in which filariform larvae develop in the bowel, invade local tissues and disseminate widely (autoinfection), occurs with immunosuppression due to steroids, lymphoma or renal transplantation. It presents with severe diarrhoea, oedema, hepatomegaly, paralytic ileus and concomitant Gram-negative sepsis. *Cryptosporidium parvum* is a self-limiting disease in healthy subjects but may cause debilitating diarrhoea in patients with AIDS; the only beneficial treatment is HAART. *Entamoeba coli* is a normal commensal. *Diphyllobothrium latum,* the fish tapeworm, may cause a macrocytic anaemia due to vitamin B12 deficiency. *T. soleum* cysterci, ingested in undercooked pork, develop into pork tapeworms in the gut. Ingestion of *T. soleum* eggs, passed out in the faeces, results in cysticercosis when the eggs hatch into invasive oncospheres which disseminate throughout the body.

Features of some protozoal infections

Organism	Transmission	Clinical features	Complications
Ascaris lumbricoides (roundworm)	Ingestion of eggs	1. Eosinophilic pneumonia during larval migration 2. Abdominal discomfort with large worm burdens	Intestinal, biliary or pancreatic obstruction by adult worms
Ankylostoma duodenale and *Necator americanus* (hookworm)	Penetration of intact skin by larvae	1. 'Ground itch' at entry site 2. Mild eosinophilic pneumonia	Iron deficiency anaemia
Trichuris trichuria (Whipworm)	Ingestion of eggs	Usually asymptomatic, heavy infection may present with bloody diarrhoea	Rectal prolapse in heavy infection

(continued)

Organism	Transmission	Clinical features	Complications
Enterobius vermicularis	Ingestion of eggs	Pruritus ani	Very rarely appendicitis
Strongyloides stercoralis	Penetration of intact skin or intestinal wall (autoinfection) by larvae	1. Skin wheals due to larval migration 'larva crurans' 2. Mild eosinophilic pneumonia	Hyper infection syndrome Gram negative septicaemia
Toxocara canis/cati	Ingestion of eggs in dog/cat faeces	Fever, hepatomegaly, eosinophilia 'visceral larva migrans'	Blindness due to ocular disease
Taenia saginata (beef tapeworm)	Ingestion of encysted larvae in undercooked beef	Asymptomatic	Rarely intestinal obstruction
Taenia soleum (pork tapeworm)	1. Ingestion of encysted larvae in undercooked pork 2. Ingestion of eggs in human faeces	1. Asymptomatic 2. Calcified tissue cysts on X-ray	Epilepsy due to tissue cysts in the brain
Echinococcus granulosus (hydatid disease)	Ingestion of eggs in dog faeces	Dependent on cyst site, e.g. filling defects and obstruction in the liver	Anaphylactic reaction following release of allergenic cyst contents
Trichinella spiralis	Ingestion of encysted larvae in undercooked meat	Fever, eosinophilia, myositis, periorbital oedema	Rarely myocarditis, encephalitis or pneumonitis
Schistosoma sp.	Eggs excreted by freshwater snails hatch into cercariae which penetrate intact skin	1. Rash at portal of entry 'Swimmers itch' 2. 'Katayama fever' characterised by eosinophilia, cough, diarrhoea, urticaria, and hepatosplenomegaly 3. Haematuria in haematobium infection 4. Bloody diarrhoea in mansoni or japonicum infection	1. Obstructive uropathy, renal stones and bladder carcinoma with haematobium 2. Periportal fibrosis, portal hypotension and cor pulmonale with mansoni and japonicum

Q 15. **Regarding HIV infection which of the following is true?**

A. AIDS dementia complex is due to JC virus reactivation
B. Time to development of AIDS is longer with HIV-2 infection than HIV-1 infection
C. Prophylaxis against *Toxoplasma gondii* should be started in patients with positive anti-*Toxoplasma* IgG and a CD4 count of $<200 \times 10^6/l$
D. *Mycobacterium avium* complex prophylaxis is best undertaken with rifabutin
E. Cervical carcinoma is an AIDS defining illness

Q 16. **A 25-year-old heterosexual man is about to begin highly active anti retroviral therapy (HAART). He is concerned about side effects. Which drugs are linked with the correct side effect?**

A. Abacavir is associated with hyperlipidaemia
B. Nevirapine is associated with lactic acidosis
C. Indinavir is associated with severe skin rash
D. Didanosine is associated with peripheral neuropathy
E. Zidovudine is associated with a microcytic anaemia

A 15. E

Invasive cervical carcinoma along with Kaposi's sarcoma and B-cell non-Hodgkin's lymphoma are malignancies currently considered AIDS defining illnesses. HIV-2 which occurs mainly in West Africa has a lower transmission rate and slower progression to AIDS than HIV-1. AIDS dementia complex which occurs in up to 50% of cases with late disease is due to the direct effect of HIV on the brain. JC virus reactivation is the cause of progressive multifocal leukoencephalopathy (PML). Prophylaxis against *Toxoplasma gondii* reactivation in seropositive individuals is initiated when the CD4 count is $<100 \times 10^6$/l. Rifabutin can be used for MAC prophylaxis but is less effective than clarithromycin or azithromycin and has numerous interaction with antiretrovirals.

A 16. D

Protease inhibitors, e.g. amprenavir, indinavir, nelfinavir, ritonavir and saquinavir are associated with hyperlipidaemia during the early course of therapy and lipodystrophy after prolonged therapy. Lactic acidosis with hepatic steatosis is a severe complication of nucleoside reverse transcriptase inhibitors (NRTI's), i.e. zidovudine, abacavir, didanosine, lamavidine, stavudine and zalcitabine. Rashes are common with non-nucleoside reverse transcriptase (nevirapine, efavirenz, delavirdine). A macrocytosis sometimes accompanied by anaemia may develop after initiation of zidovudine therapy, peripheral neuropathy is an important side effect of didanosine therapy and may occur with other NRTI's

AIDS defining illnesses
The following are diagnostic of AIDS even without laboratory evidence of HIV infection
- Oesophageal or pulmonary candidiasis
- Extra pulmonary cryptococcal disease
- Disseminated CMV
- Cryptosporodial diarrhoea <1 month
- Oesophageal HSV or mucocutaneous HSV ulceration persisting >1 month
- Kaposi's sarcoma
- Cerebral lymphoma
- Disseminated MAC
- PCP pneumonia
- PML
- Cerebral toxoplasmosis

Prophylaxis for opportunistic disease in HIV (Infectious Diseases Society of America Guidelines)

Organism	Indication	1st choice	Alternative
Pneumocystis carinii	CD4 count <200 × 10⁶/l Previous PCP	Co-trimoxazole	Dapsone +/− pyrimethamine Nebulised pentamadine Atovaquone
Toxoplasma gondii	CD4 count <100 × 10⁶/l and anti-Toxoplasma IgG +ve	Co-trimoxazole	Dapsone + pyrimethamine
Mycobacterium tuberculosis	Previous TB or contact with active case	Isoniazid + pyridoxine for 12 months	Rifampicin + pyrazinamide for 2 months
Mycobacterium avium complex	CD4 count <50 × 10⁶/l	Clarithromycin or azithromycin	Rifabutin
Streptococcus pneumoniae	All patients	Pneumococcal vaccine	–
*Hepatitis B	Negative Hep B serology, high risk of infection	Hepatitis B vaccine	–
*Bacterial infections	Neutropenia	G-CSF/GM-CSF	–
*Candidiasis/ Cryptococcosis	CD4 count <50 × 10⁶/l	Fluconazole	–

* Should be considered on a case by case basis, G-CSF, granulocyte colony-stimulating factor, GM-CSF, granulocyte macrophage colony stimulating factor.

Diarrhoeal Syndromes

Q 17. A 75-year-old woman with abdominal cramps and bloody diarrhoea is prescribed ciprofloxacin by her GP. She is admitted to hospital 3 days later with a right sided hemiparesis. Temperature 37.5°C, Hb 8.6 g/dl, WBC 16.6 × 10⁹/l, platelets 57 × 10⁹/l, PT, APPT and INR normal, urea 23.6 mmol/l; creatinine 287 mmol/l. Examination of a peripheral blood film reveals many fragmented red blood cells. Which organism is the most likely cause of these abnormalities?

A. Enteroinvasive *E. coli*
B. *Campylobacter jejuni*
C. *Salmonella enteritidis*
D. Verotoxigenic *E. coli*
E. *Shigella flexneri*

Q 18. Which of the following statements is true?

A. Piperacillin/tazobactam therapy is a common cause of antibiotic associated diarrhoea
B. Diarrhoea due to *Vibrio cholerae* is accompanied by marked fever
C. There is an association between antibiotic associated diarrhoea and *Clostridium perfringens*
D. *Staphylococcus aureus* causes an invasive enteritis
E. Norwalk agent causes a self-limiting bloody diarrhoea

A 17. D

The presentation and blood abnormalities are typical of the haemolytic uraemic syndrome (HUS) and thrombotic thrombocytopenic purpura (TTP). This may develop after infection with verotoxigen (also known as enterohaemorrhagic) *E. coli*; usually but not exclusively serotype 0157:H7. Antibiotic therapy may predispose to the development of HUS and is not recommended. Enteroinvasive *E. coli*, *C. jejuni*, *Salmonella enteritidis* and *Shigella flexneri* may all cause bloody diarrhoea but only *Shigella dysentariae* serotype 1 which produces a Shiga toxin has been associated with HUS.

A 18. C

Antibiotic associated diarrhoea (AAD) is commonest after exposure to broad spectrum antibiotics especially cephalosporins, amoxicillin and clindamycin. Piperacillin/tazobactam (along with quinolones and aminoglycosides) only rarely causes AAD, probably because of its limited penetration into the gut lumen. AAD is most commonly due to overgrowth of toxigenic strains of *Clostridium difficile* but *Clostridium perfringens* and *Staphylococcus aureus* have also been identified as possible causative organisms. *Vibrio cholerae* causes severe secretary diarrhoea without fever. Food poisoning due to *Staphylococcus aureus* is due to local action of staphylococcal enterotoxin ingested in contaminated food. Norwalk agent causes epidemic vomiting and diarrhoea without blood.

Gastroenteritis
- Causes: i. Secretary diarrhoea; *S. aureus,* Enterotoxigenic *E. coli, Clostridium perfringens, V. cholerae, B. cereus,* viruses (SRSV, adenovirus, calicivirus, Norwalk). ii. Invasive enteritis: *Shigellae, Salmonellae, Campylobacter jejuni,* enteroinvasive *E. coli,* verotoxigenic *E. coli, Yersinia enterocolitica, V. parahaemolyticus, Giardia lamblia*
- Oral rehydration is the mainstay of treatment; antibiotics are indicated for *Giardia* and bacteraemic infections, e.g. *Salmonella* and *Shigella* once pathogens have been cultured
- Empirical therapy should be limited to 'high risk' cases: age <5 or >60 years, immunodeficiency, gastric hypochlorhydria, inflammatory bowel disease, valvular heart disease, prosthetic valve, aortic aneurysm, diabetes mellitus, renal impairment, RA, SLE
- Avoid antimotility agents

Haemolytic uraemic syndrome (HUS)/Thrombotic thrombocytopenic purpura (TTP)
- Caused by Shiga toxin producing verocytotoxigenic *E. coli* and *S. dysentariae.* Some drugs, e.g. quinine, cycosporin A, ticlopidine and cisplatin have also been implicated

- Shiga toxin binds to Gb$_3$ gycolipid receptors in microvasculature, causes local cytokine release and inflammation
- Presents with abdominal pain, bloody diarrhoea, lack of fever and complications of TTP, i.e. anaemia and focal neurological signs
- Investigations may show ↑WBC, ↓Hb, fragmented RBC's on blood film, ↓platelets and albumin, ↑urea, creatinine and LDH. Coagulation studies are usually normal
- Verotoxigenic organisms or *E. coli* 0157 may be identified in faeces or food
- Treatment includes fluid resuscitation and plasma exchange. Platelet transfusions should be avoided unless there is life threatening bleeding as they may provoke cerebral or myocardial infarction

Bloodstream Infections

Q 19. Blood cultures drawn peripherally and via a non-tunnelled central line from a febrile patient on the ITU grow *Staphylococcus aureus*. Which of the following is the most appropriate action?

    A. Remove the central venous cannula and reassess at 48 h
    B. Remove the cannula and perform a transoesophageal echocardiogram
    C. Commence IV flucloxacillin and reassess at 48 h
    D. Send swabs from the cannula site for culture
    E. Commence antibiotic lock therapy with vancomycin

Q 20. With respect to the sepsis syndrome which of the following statements is false?

    A. Bactericidal/permeability – increasing protein binds lipopolysaccharide
    B. Plasma lactate levels are greatly elevated
    C. Corticosteroids are of proven benefit
    D. Recombinant human activated protein C reduces mortality in severe sepsis
    E. Elevation of serum procalcitonin is a specific marker of bacterial infection

A 19. B

Culture of the same organism from peripheral and central blood cultures is indicative of catheter related bloodstream infection (CRBSI). Culture of $>10^2$ cfu from the catheter tip in a febrile patient also implies CRSBI; swabs from the cannula site are unhelpful. *S. aureus* bacteraemia is associated with a high incidence of complications, e.g. endocarditis and osteomyelitis and excess mortality unless all intravascular devices are removed and antimicrobial therapy commenced. As the duration of therapy is dependent on the presence or absence of metastatic complications an echocardiogram is recommended in all patients. In contrast CRBSI due to coagulase negative staphylococci can often be treated with antibiotic lock (agent instilled into lumen of line) or short course vancomycin therapy thus preserving the line.

A 20. C

In Gram negative sepsis lipopolysaccharide (LPS) activates multiple inflammatory cytokines by binding to LPS-binding protein and CD14. Bactericidal/permeability – increasing protein, released from neutrophils, preferentially binds LPS and acts as an anti-inflammatory molecule. Lactate levels are elevated up to 7 fold in severe sepsis, reflecting tissue hypoxia, and are a useful in monitoring response to therapy. Steroids are effective in animal models if given prior to the onset of sepsis, but meta-analysis of trials conducted in humans shows no benefit whatsoever. Recombinant human activated protein C (Drotrecogin alfa) inhibits thrombosis and inflammation. It has been shown to reduce mortality from sepsis in a large randomised trial, although there were significantly more episodes of severe bleeding in the treated group. It has been approved in the USA as an adjunctive treatment for severe sepsis. Procalcitonin is elevated in bacterial sepsis and correlates with the degree of severity; unlike C-reactive protein it is not elevated in the systemic inflammatory response syndrome due to non-infectious causes, e.g. pancreatitis, trauma, and burns.

Management of IV cannula related infections (Infectious Diseases Society of America)
Non-tunnelled devices

- *Staphylococcus aureus*: Remove device, 14 days systemic therapy, extended to 4–6 weeks if TEE +ve
- Coagulase negative staphylococci: Remove device and treat with systemic therapy for 5–7 days OR retain device and treat with systemic +/– antibiotic lock therapy for 10–14 days
- Gram negative infection: Remove device, 10–14 days systemic therapy
- *Candida*: Remove device, systemic antifungal therapy for 14 days after the last +ve culture

Tunnelled or implanted devices

- Remove if the patient is severely ill or there are complications, e.g. endocarditis, tunnel infection or septic thrombosis
- Consider antibiotic lock therapy with appropriate antibiotic

Definitions of sepsis

- Sepsis: temp <36°C or >38°C, pulse >90/min, resp rate >20 with a presumed site of infection
- Severe sepsis = sepsis with organ dysfunction (hypotension, oliguria, confusion, lactic acidosis)
- Septic shock = severe sepsis with hypotension despite adequate fluid resuscitation
- Bacteraemia = bacteria present in the blood as confirmed by culture, may be transient and present with or without sepsis

Sexually Transmitted Infections

Q 21. A 42-year-old man recently arrived from Ghana is referred to you in the STD clinic with urethral discharge. Which organism is least likely to cause this?

A. *Calymmatobacterium granulomatis*
B. *Neisseria gonorrhoea*
C. *Chlamydia trachomatis*
D. *Ureaplasma urealyticum*
E. *Trichomonas vaginalis*

Q 22. Which of the following statements is true regarding syphilis?

A. Gummata are found in secondary syphilis
B. The VDRL remains strongly positive after successful treatment of primary syphilis
C. The primary chancre of syphilis is tender
D. Treatment of neurosyphilis in a patient with penicillin allergy is with doxycycline
E. The CSF should be examined in a patient with HIV and syphilis co-infection

[A] 21. A

Calymmatobacterium granulomatis is a Gram negative organism that causes granuloma inguinale (donovanosis). The disease is endemic in Southern India and also found in Africa, the Caribbean and South America. It presents as a painless ulcer on the prepuce or labia.

[A] 22. E

Gummata, granulomatous lesions in the skin and soft tissues, are a feature of tertiary syphilis. The VDRL titre falls after successful treatment, reappearance or a rise in titre suggests relapse or reinfection. For penicillin allergic patients doxycycline is a useful alternative for primary, secondary, latent and cardiovascular or gummatous tertiary syphilis. Patients with neurosyphilis should be desensitised to penicillin as no other active agent achieves adequate concentration in the CSF. Patients with syphilis and HIV should have a lumbar puncture and be treated for neurosyphilis regardless of the stage of the disease.

Serological tests for syphilis
Non-treponemal tests (detect non-specific antibodies to lipoidal antigens)
- VDRL (Venereal diseases reference laboratory)
- RPR (Rapid plasma regain)
- Become +ve 1–4 weeks after development of primary chancre
- Titre correlates with activity of disease
- False +ve occur in pregnancy, old age, other spirochaetal infections, TB, malaria, HIV, toxoplasmosis, acute bacterial infection, SLE, polyarteritis nodosa, RA, primary biliary cirrhosis, ITP, malignancy and malnutrition

Treponemal tests (detect specific antibodies to treponemal antigens)
- FTA-ABS (Fluorescent treponemal antibody test)
- TPHA (*Treponema pallidum* haemaugglutination assay)
- EIA (IgG or IgM enzyme immunoassay)

	VDRL	TPHA
Primary syphilis	Positive in 70%	Positive in 90%
Secondary syphilis	Positive high titre	Positive
Latent syphilis	Positive titre falls with time	Positive
Neurosyphilis	Negative or low titre	Positive

Bone and Joint Infection

Q 23. As the rheumatology SHO you are asked to see a 54 yr old man with a tender swollen left knee. Which of the following statements is true?

A. In previously healthy adults over 80% of cases of bacterial arthritis are due to *Staphylococcus aureus*
B. In acute septic arthritis a Gram stain of synovial fluid is positive in >90% of cases
C. Hepatitis C virus is associated with a monoarticular arthritis
D. Reactive arthritis is most common in HLA-B27 negative patients
E. Disseminated gonococcal arthritis presents with migratory polyarthralgias, tenosynovitis and dermatitis

Q 24. A 42-year-old man presents with arthralgia and a skin rash. Which of the following is *not* a likely diagnosis?

A. Lyme disease
B. Syphilis
C. Rat bite fever
D. Lymphogranuloma venereum
E. Dengue fever

A 23. **B**

S. aureus is the cause of 40% of cases of septic arthritis overall and for 80% of cases in diabetics or those with rheumatoid arthritis. The triad of migratory polyarthralgia, tenosynovitis and dermatitis are characteristic of disseminated gonococcal arthritis. Synovial fluid culture is positive in 90% of cases of non-gonococcal bacterial arthritis, the Gram stain in only 50%. In gonococcal arthritis the organism is most readily isolated from genitourinary cultures (70–90%), synovial fluid is positive by Gram's stain in 10% and culture in 25%. Hepatitis C can cause a symmetric polyarthritis that is often accompanied by a positive rheumatoid factor thus being confused with rheumatoid arthritis. HLA-B27 is associated with an increased incidence of reactive arthritis especially after gastrointestinal infections with *Shigella flexneri*, *Salmonella enteritridis*, *S. typhimurium*, *Y. enterecolitica* and *C. jejuni*.

A 24. **D**

Lymphogranuloma venereum is associated with a reactive oligoarticular arthritis but no rash. Erythema migrans and arthralgias occur in early disseminated lyme disease, joint pains accompany the maculopapular rash of secondary syphilis. Rat bite fever due to *Streptobacillus moniliformis* is a septicaemic disease following a rat bite or exposure to contaminated milk. There is a maculopapular or petechial rash, arthritis of large joints, abscesses and rarely endocarditis. Muscular pain and arthralgia (breakbone fever) and a maculopapular rash on the trunk occur in Dengue fever syndrome.

Septic arthritis
- Usually occurs secondary to haematogenous seeding during bacteraemia
- Risk factors; RA, crystal arthropathy, OA, IVDU
- Acute monoarthritis is septic until proven otherwise
- Organisms; *S. aureus,* streptococci, coliforms (IVDU's)
- Disseminated gonococcal infection (DGI) presents with migratory polyarthralgia, tenosynovitis and dermatitis, 3 times more common in women
- DGI responds rapidly to antibiotics in 1–3 days, other organisms need prolonged treatment 3–4 weeks

Reiter's syndrome
- Syndrome of arthritis, conjunctivitis and urethritis following bacterial infection
- Commoner in males, 80% HLA-B27 +ve
- Acute asymmetrical polyarthritis occurs up to 4 weeks after infection
- Strong association with *C. trachomatis, Salmonella, Shigella* and *Yersinia* infections

Osteomyelitis

- Acute osteomyelitis usually haematogenously spread and affects metaphyses of long bones. Contiguous spread from local soft tissue infection occurs in open fractures and sacral pressure sores
- Organisms; *S. aureus,* Group B streptococci (neonates), *Salmonella* (sickle cell disease), coliforms and *pseudomonas* (elderly)
- Consider vertebral osteomyelitis in an elderly patient with back pain and raised ESR
- Treatment includes long term antibiotic therapy and surgical debridement of dead bone (sequestrum)

Infections in Compromised Hosts

Q 25. A patient with acute myeloid leukaemia has a bone marrow transplantation. Which of the following is true?

    A. Following bone marrow transplantation the risk of CMV disease is highest when the donor is seropositive

    B. Ganciclovir is effective in reducing mortality from CMV pneumonitis

    C. A bone marrow transplant patient in contact with chickenpox should be given acyclovir prophylaxis

    D. CMV disease following bone marrow transplantation commonly presents as retinitis

    E. Respiratory syncytial virus pneumonia may be prevented by ribavirin therapy

Q 26. In a young patient with previous splenectomy after a road traffic accident which of the following is false:

    A. There is an increased risk of severe malaria

    B. Lifelong penicillin prophylaxis is recommended

    C. Meningococcal vaccination is recommended in the UK

    D. Pneumococcal infection carries a mortality of up to 60%

    E. There is an increased risk of infection with *Capnocytophaga canimorsus*

A 25. E

In bone marrow transplantation (BMT) the risk of CMV disease is highest when the recipient is seropositive in contrast to solid organ transplantation when donor seropositivity represents the highest risk. CMV commonly causes pneumonia following BMT, it very rarely causes retinitis. Although ganciclovir is often given for CMV disease there is little evidence of its efficacy, only when combined with normal immunoglobulin is there a slight reduction in mortality. A BMT patient exposed to chickenpox or herpes zoster should be screened for VZV IgG antibody and if negative given varicella zoster immunoglobulin (VZIG). Treatment of RSV upper respiratory tract infection with ribavirin may prevent the development of RSV pneumonia.

A 26. C

Although patients with dysfunctional spleens are at increased risk of meningococcal infection the current vaccine is not active against group B strains prevalent in the UK. Immunisation with A and C vaccine is only recommended for travelers to endemic areas.

Infections in patients with dysfunction spleen
- Increased risk of *S. pneumoniae, H. influenzae, N. meningitides,* severe malaria, *Capnocytophaga canimorsus* (from dog bites) and babesiosis
- Patients should be vaccinated against *S. pneumoniae, H. influenzae* and influenza
- Lifelong antibiotic prophylaxis with penicillin, amoxicillin or erythromycin is recommended

Infections in bone marrow transplant patients
- Myeloablative chemotherapy leads to prolonged neutropenia (~21 days) and mucositis. Bacterial and fungal infection occur and episodes of febrile neutropenia are treated with pre-emptive antibiotics and antifungals
- After engraftment acute graft versus host disease (GVHD) with rash and hepatic dysfunction may develop, interstitial pneumonia due to CMV, PCP, adenovirus and *Aspergillus* may occur
- Bacterial infections and chronic GVHD continue to affect those on long term immunosuppression

Infections in solid organ transplant patients
- Risk is highest during 1st year and those given antirejection treatment
- Infections follow a predictable course
- 1st month: Nosocomial pneumonia and wound infection, IV cannula infections, reactivation of strongyloides and tuberculosis
- 1st 6 months: CMV, VZV, HSV, aspergillosis, *Pneumocystis carinii, Toxoplasma gondii*
- >6 months: Progressive viral infections, *Nocardia asteroides,* community acquired pneumonia

Central Nervous System Infections

Q 27. **A 12-year-old girl presents with fever, headache and a maculopapular rash. Meningococcal sepsis is suspected. Which of the following is true?**

    A. Blood cultures are unhelpful

    B. Chloramphenicol is the drug of choice in patients with previous anaphylaxis to penicillins

    C. Patients treated with ceftriaxone require rifampicin prophylaxis to eradicate carriage

    D. *N. meningitidis* can be isolated from throat swabs in 90% of cases

    E. A SHO who performed a lumbar puncture on a confirmed case will require prophylactic antibiotics

Q 28. **Which statement is true of viral encephalitis?**

    A. Transmission of West Nile encephalitis involves a tick vector

    B. Rabies encephalitis occurs following haematogenous spread of the virus from a bite wound

    C. CT scanning is the imaging mode of choice

    D. Herpes simplex encephalitis is associated with a high mortality

    E. Electroencephalogram (EEG) changes in the frontal lobes suggest herpes simplex encephalitis

A 27. **B**

Chloramphenicol has good activity against *N. meningitidis*, *S. pneumoniae* and *H. influenzae* and is recommended as the treatment of choice for patients with anaphylaxis to penicillins in the 'UK consensus statement on the diagnosis and treatment of bacterial meningitis'. Bacteraemia often accompanies meningococcal meningitis and the organism can be isolated from blood cultures, the yield is reduced by prior administration of antibiotics. Ceftriaxone reliably eradicates throat carriage of *N. meningitides*, therefore only patients who are NOT treated with ceftriaxone require treatment with rifampicin. *N. meningitidis* can be isolated from throat swabs in 50% of cases. Prophylactic antibiotics are only required for medical staff who have had mucosal contact with the patients respiratory secretions, e.g. mouth to mouth resuscitation.

A 28. **D**

Untreated HSV encephalitis has a mortality of 80% acyclovir treatment reduces this to approximately 25%. MRI scanning is more sensitive than CT and is the investigation of choice. West Nile virus found in Uganda, Egypt and Israel and now emerging in the Eastern USA, is transmitted to humans from animals via a mosquito vector. Rabies virus reaches the CNS via a myoneuronal route. After local replication at the bite wound, the virus spreads by anterograde and retrograde axonal transport along peripheral nerves to the brainstem and limbic system. EEG changes in the temporal lobes are strongly suggestive of HSV encephalitis.

Encephalitis
Acute
- DNA viruses; HSV, CMV, EBV, VZV, HHV-6, adenovirus
- Enteroviruses; Coxsackie, ECHO, polio
- Flaviviruses: Japanese B, St. Louis, West Nile, Tick borne encephalitis
- Bunyaviruses: California encephalitis, La Crosse
- Togaviruses: Western equine encephalitis, Eastern equine encephalitis

Post infectious
- Viral infections: Mumps, rubella, VZV, HSV, Influenza
- Bacterial infections: *Mycoplasma, S. pyogenes, Campylobacter*
- Vaccines: Measles, rabies, oral polio, Japanese B

New Antimicrobials

Q 29. Which statement is true concerning linezolid?

A. It is an inhibitor of monoamine oxidase
B. It is a cell wall active agent
C. It has no activity against Gram negative bacteria
D. It is rapidly bactericidal
E. It is superior to vancomycin in the treatment of MRSA pneumonia and soft tissue infection

Q 30. Which statement is true concerning Quinupristin/dalfopristin?

A. It has excellent activity against *Enterococcus faecalis*
B. It is a combination of ketolide antibiotics
C. It is excreted predominantly in the urine
D. It is an inhibitor of hepatic cytochrome P450
E. It should be administered via a peripheral vein

A 29. A

Linezolid is an oxazolidonone antibiotic acting on bacterial protein synthesis by inhibiting formation of a 70s initiation complex. It is highly active against Gram positive bacteria, but In-vitro also has limited activity against *Haemophilus influenzae* and *Moraxella catarrhalis* (MIC 4–16 mg/l), other Gram negative bacteria are resistant via efflux mechanisms. It is bacteriostatic and synergy has not been observed with any other antimicrobial agent. In phase III trials, linezolid therapy was equivalent to flucloxacillin or clarithromycin therapy in soft tissue infections, and to vancomycin with aztreonam therapy in nosocomial pneumonia. In-vitro, linezolid has monoamine oxidase inhibitor activity; patients should avoid tyramine containing foods to eliminate the risk of a hypertensive reaction.

A 30. D

Quinupristin/dalfopristin is the first injectable streptogrammin. It is active against Gram positive bacteria including *Staphylococci*, *Streptococci* and *Enterococcus faecium*. It is not active against *Enterococcus faecalis*. The combination is bactericidal against strains sensitive to macrolides. In the presence of macrolide resistance the drug is only bacteriostatic as the quinupristin activity of the combination is lost. The drug is excreted primarily in the bile and is a hepatic enzyme inhibitor. Due to thrombophlebitis and pain at the infusion site the drug should be given via a central vein.

Linezolid
- Synthetic oxazolidonone antibiotic with novel mechanism of action on early protein synthesis binds to 50s ribosome and prevents formation of 70s initiation complex
- Highly active against Gram positive organisms including MRSA, VRE and GISA (gylcopeptide intermediate *Staphylococcus aureus*) strains
- Licensed in UK for Gram positive pneumonia and complicated soft tissue infections
- Almost 100% oral bioavailability
- Prolonged courses (>14 days) have been associated with thrombocytopenia due to reversible marrow suppression, FBC should be monitored
- Resistance in *Enterococci* and *S. aureus* was seen within months of its introduction

Quinupristin/dalfopristin
- Combination of a group B and group A streptogrammin
- Inhibits protein synthesis by blocking aminoacyl-tRNA complexes binding to the ribosome (quinupristin) and inhibiting peptide bond formation (dalfopristin)
- Active against most Gram positive bacteria except *E. faecalis*
- Equivalent to vancomycin in skin and soft tissue infections and nosocomial pneumonia
- Useful for severe infection with vancomycin resistant *Enterococcus faecium*
- Adverse effects include arthralgia (10% of patients) and thrombophlebitis

Infectious Diseases

New Antimicrobials

Nephrology

Renal Vascular Diseases

Q 1. A 33-year-old man with hard-to-control hypertension is found to have unilateral renal artery stenosis. The following statements about renal artery stenosis are true except:

A. 80% of the cases are due to atherosclerosis
B. Fibromuscular dysplasia commonly affects young men
C. Hypokalaemia and metabolic alkalosis may occur
D. Renovascular hypertension due to fibromuscular dysplasia responds to revascularisation in the majority of patients
E. May produce an epigastric bruit

Q 2. A 2-year-old boy with severe diarrhoea presents to the emergency department with oliguria, fever, chills and pain in the flanks. Examination revealed severe dehydration, lumbar tenderness, right kidney was palpable and tender. The blood pressure was 100/40. Urine examination revealed haematuria and proteinuria. Serum urea and creatinine were raised. Serum albumin was normal. Cbc and peripheral smear appear normal. The most probable diagnosis is:

A. Post streptococcal glomerulonephritis
B. Nephrotic syndrome
C. Haemolytic uremic syndrome
D. Renal vein thrombosis
E. Septic shock

Q 3. A 20-year-old afrocarribean man has impaired renal function and sickle cell disease. He is at risk of developing all the following except:

A. Papillary necrosis
B. Nephrogenic diabetes insipidus
C. Focal segmental glomerulo sclerosis
D. Hyperuricemia
E. Membranoproliferative glomerulonephritis

A 1. B

Renal artery stenosis accounts for about 5% of cases of hypertension. 90% of cases are due to atherosclerosis, commonly affecting the proximal part and the ostium of the renal artery. These people also have commonly other stigmata of atherosclerosis, like peripheral vascular disease, myocardial infarction, etc. Fibromuscular dysplasia, a rare cause of renal artery stenosis, usually affects the distal part of the renal artery and is commonly found in young women. It produces a string of beads appearance in angiography. Dysplasia commonly affects the media of the artery. Hypokalaemia and metabolic alkalosis may occur due to the compensatory hyperaldosteronism. Hypertension due to FMD usually responds to revascularisation better than atherosclerosis induced hypertension. Balloon angioplasty is the preferred procedure. An epigastric bruit may be auscultatable in renal artery stenosis.

A 2. D

Acute glomerulonephritis commonly presents with oliguric acute renal failure, usually 2 weeks after a throat or skin infection. Oedema and hypertension are predominant features. RBC casts are present. Nephrotic syndrome is not usually associated with fever and nephrotic range proteinuria is the rule. The HUS is a microangiopathic haemolytic anaemia with predominant renal involvement, usually follows infection by *E.coli* o157:h7. Peripheral smear shows fragmented RBCs in the majority of cases. Good prognosis in children. Thrombotic thrombocytopenic purpura is a similar syndrome affecting adults with predominant neurologic involvement. For both cases coagulation profile is normal, but thrombocytopenia is present. Renal vein thrombosis can present as an acute problem in children usually following dehydration with fever, lumbar pain, etc. Treatment is with anti-coagulation. Septic shock usually does not produce lumbar tenderness and enlarged unilateral kidney.

A 3. E

Sickle cell nephropathy produces ischaemic injury due to sickling in the hypoxic medullary vasculature. It also produces hyperfiltration injury due to the associated anaemia and due to the changes in glomerular pore radius and number. Papillary necrosis results due to the medullary ischaemia. It presents with fever, loin pain, haematuria. Ring shadow is appreciated on pyelography. Nephrogenic diabetes insipidus is due to the medullary ischaemia affecting the tubular epithelium concentrating ability. Defective purine excretion coupled with increased production from the bone marrow account for the hyperuricemia. FSGS is a common end result of all conditions producing hyperfiltration injury, e.g. diabetes mellitus, compensatory hyperfiltration. MPGN is not associated with sickle cell disease.

Causes of renal vein thrombosis
- Trauma
- Oral contraceptive use
- Dehydration
- Renal cell carcinoma
- Extrinsic compression (lymph nodes, aneurysm, tumour)
- Nephrotic syndrome
- Pregnancy
- Hypercoagulable states

Causes of papillary necrosis: usually bilateral
- Diabetes
- Sickle cell disease
- Pyelonephritis
- Chronic alcoholism
- Vascular insufficiency

Renal Anatomy and Physiology

Q 4. The following are true regarding renal absorption of solutes except:

A. Glucose and sodium are co-transported in the proximal tubular cell by sglt 1

B. Renal splay diminishes the renal threshold for glucose

C. Amino acids and phosphate are reabsorbed by secondary active transport

D. Fanconi's syndrome has as its components renal tubular acidosis and phosphaturia

E. Glomerular filtrate becomes more dilute as it passes down the descending loop of Henle

F. $Na^+ K^+ 2Cl^-$ transporter is situated in the ascending loop of Henle

Q 5. Which of the following statements is true?

A. Renal blood flow is around 15% of the cardiac output

B. Sympathetic stimulation decreases renin secretion from the juxtaglomerular apparatus

C. Renal medullary blood flow is much less compared to the renal cortex

D. Capillary pericytes are a part of juxtaglomerular apparatus

E. Renal filtration fraction is around 0.5

A 5.   C

Sodium is reabsorbed along its concentration gradient into the tubular cell and by active transport from there to the interstitial fluid. Substances like glucose, aminoacids, phosphate, H^+, etc are linked to the active transport of Na^+ and are reabsorbed by secondary active transport. Water follows down the concentration gradient by aquaphorin 1 channel in the proximal convoluted channel. sglt 1 and 2 are sodium glucose transporters found in renal tubules. Renal threshold for glucose is predicted as 300 mg/dl, but because of the differences in absorption rates by different nephrons the actual observed value is around 180–200 mg/dl. This difference in reabsorption capacities leads to the renal splay observed in actual glucose reabsorption curve. Descending limb of Henle's loop is permeable to water and relatively impermeable to the solutes. So filtrate becomes more concentrated as it passes down the loop of Henle descending limb. Fanconi's syndrome is a disorder of the proximal tubule characterised by glucosuria, phosphaturia, aminoaciduria, rta type 1, uricosuria, etc. It can be either congenital or acquired. $Na^+k^+2cl^-$ transporter is the transporter present in the ascending loop of Henle. Renal blood flow is around 20–25% of cardiac output. Renal medullary blood flow is less compared to the cortical flow and thus medulla is more prone for ischaemia. Sympathetic stimulation improves renin release from juxtaglomerular (JG) apparatus by beta1 receptor stimulation. Juxtaglomerular apparatus is formed by macula densa cells modified from the tubular epithelium, JG cells from the afferent arteriole and lacis cells from the mesangium. Renal filtration fraction – the ratio of glomerular filtration rate (GFR) to renal plasma flow is around 16–20.

Causes of Fanconi's syndrome
- Congenital – dominant, recessive or x linked
- Wilson's disease
- Galactosaemia
- Tyrosinaemia
- Cystinosis
- Fructose intolerance
- Lowes oculocerebral syndrome
- Multiple myeloma
- Amyloid
- Heavy metal toxicity

Acute Renal Failure (ARF) and Management

Q 6. A 50-year-old male patient presents with oliguria and swelling of legs to the emergency room. He gives history of diarrhoea for 5 days and looks dehydrated. Which of the following tests suggests prerenal ARF as the diagnosis?

A. Fractional extraction of sodium >2
B. Renal failure index <1
C. Urinary sodium >20
D. Muddy brown urinary casts
E. Proteinuria mild

Q 7. A 40-year-old woman is admitted with elevated creatinine and a history of being unwell for only one week. Which of the following finding would be least consistent with a diagnosis of Acute Renal Failure?

A. Anaemia
B. Bleeding manifestations
C. Hyperkalaemia
D. Vigorous diuresis
E. Bilateral contracted kidneys on ultrasound

Q 8. The following are true about urinalysis except:

A. Dipstick is more sensitive for the detection of myeloma proteins than sulphosalicylic acid technique
B. Broad casts are suggestive of Chronic Renal Failure (CRF) due to any cause
C. Hyaline casts may be a normal component of urine
D. Prerenal ARF presents with a bland urinary sediment
E. Eosinophiluria may be present in cholesterol embolisation of the kidney

A 6. **B**

A 7. **E**

A 8. **A**

Analysis of urine and blood biochemistry is useful in distinguishing prerenal ARF from acute tubular necrosis.

Diagnostic Index	Prerenal ARF	Intrinsic renal ARF
Fractional sodium excretion (ratio of Na clearance to Cr clearance)	<1	>1
Urine sodium concentration	≤10	≥20
Urine specific gravity	>1.020	~1.010
Renal failure index	<1	>1
Urine osmolality	≥500	~300

Prerenal ARF is usually associated with a bland urinary sediment while intrinsic renal failure or ATN (Acute Tubular Necrosis) are associated with a muddy brown granular casts in the urine. Proteinuria may be a part of both prerenal ARF or renal ARF. Mild anaemia is a part of ARF due to impaired erythropoiesis, haemolysis, etc. Bleeding manifestations can occur in ARF due to thrombasthenia due to the uremic toxins especially guanidino succinic acid. Hyperkalaemia commonly complicates ARF due to the tubular dysfunction preventing K^+ excretion. Vigorous diuresis can be a part of the recovery phase of intrinsic ARF. Bilateral contracted kidneys usually suggest chronic renal failure. Dipstick method usually has a sensitivity range of 20–30 mg/dl, detects albumin readily and is less sensitive to myeloma proteins which are more readily detected by sulphosalicylic acid method or urinary electrophoresis. Hyaline casts may be a normal finding due to the excretion of tommhorsfall protein. Broad casts in urine suggests tubular dilatation and atrophy usually due to CRF. Eosinophiluria is usually seen with interstitial nephritis especially allergic. It is also a common finding in cholesterol embolisation of the kidney.

Drugs causing renal failure

1 – Drugs commonly causing prerenal ARF
- NSAIDs
- ACE inhibitors
- Antihypertensives

2 – Drugs producing acute tubular necrosis
- Radiocontrast agents
- Cyclosporine
- Antibiotics
- Cisplatin
- Ethylene glycol
- Acetaminophen
- Ticlopidine

3 – Drugs producing interstitial nephritis
- β lactams
- Trimethoprim
- Sulphonamides
- Rifampicin
- NSAIDs
- Diuretics
- Captopril
- Gold salts

Chronic Renal Failure (CRF) and Management

Q 9. **Which of the following is correct regarding CRF?**

A. Hyperkalaemia is usually not evident in otherwise uncomplicated CRF unless GFR falls to below 20 ml/min

B. Cyclosporine commonly produces hypokalaemia in post transplant patients

C. Metabolic alkalosis commonly produces hyperkalaemia

D. Intravenous erythropoietin achieves the target haemoglobin at a lower dose than subcutaneous erythropoietin

E. Dialysis dementia is usually observed with first few dialysis sittings

Q 10. **All of the following are true regarding renal osteodystrophy except:**

A. Osteitis fibrosa cystica is the most common type of renal osteodystrophy

B. Ruggerjersey spine may be seen in patients with renal osteodystrophy

C. Aluminium toxicity is a recognised cause for the osteomalacia seen in patients with CRF

D. Adynamic bone disease is associated with hyperparathyroidism

E. Phosphate restriction is essential for management of these patients

Q 11. **Which of the following is primarily responsible for the impaired platelet function in CRF?**

A. Parathyroid hormone

B. Urea

C. Creatinine

D. Guanidinosuccinic acid

E. Phosphate

A 9. **A**

A 10. **D**

A 11. **D**

Serum potassium is usually maintained till the end stages of CRF and begin to rise only after the GFR has fallen below 10 ml/min (Harrison-15th ed). Hypokalaemia can also occur due to decreased dietary intake, Fanconi's syndrome, tubular diseases, renal tubular acidosis, etc. Cyclosporine is a common cause of renal toxicity and hyperkalaemia in post transplant patients. In metabolic alkalosis, cells exchange H^+ ions with extra cellular fluid K^+ resulting in relative hypokalaemia, as a part of compensation. Erythropoietin therapy is the ideal way to treat anaemia associated with CRF. It should be combined with adequate iron and folic acid supplementation. Subcutaneous route has a sparing effect, the target haematocrit reached at a lower dose than the IV route. Dialysis dementia is a sequelae of chronic dialysis and is linked to aluminium toxicity as a potential cause. Dialysis disequilibrium is usually seen with the first few dialysis due to rapid reduction of blood urea levels.

Types of renal osteodystrophy
1 – Osteitis fibrosa cystica (50%)
  – due to POU↑, so Cu^{2+}↓
  – also PTH↑, 1,25 D_3↓
  – associated with Ca^{2+}↓, POU↑, PTH↑, AP↑
2 – Adynamic (25%)
  – Too much Ca/VITD gives, suppressive PTH
  – Additional Al toxicity/hypogonadism
3 – Osteomalacia (7%)
4 – Mixed
  – Partly 1,25 D_3↓
  – Partly Al, Fe toxicity
Ruggerjersey spine may be seen with renal bone disease. Phosphate binding with preferably calcium carbonate or acetate and desferoxamine for aluminium chelation are used for treatment of renal osteodystrophy.

Platelet disorder in CRF is usually a functional dysfunction related to the guanidinosuccinic acid blocking platelet factor 3 activation with ADP.

Drugs causing hyperkalaemia
1. ACE inhibitors
2. Amiloride
3. Cyclosporine
4. Cytotoxics
5. Heparin
6. Lithium
7. NSAIDs
8. Pentamidine
9. Spironolactone

Renal Replacement Therapy/Renal Transplantation

Q 12. A 50-year-old man on chronic haemodialysis suffers recurrent hypotension on dialysis. All the following may help except:

A. Stopping ultrafiltration
B. Isotonic saline infusion
C. Warming the dialysate
D. Salt free albumin infusion
E. Avoiding heavy meals on the day of dialysis

Q 13. The following are true of renal replacement therapy except:

A. Tenchkoff catheter is commonly used for peritoneal dialysis
B. In nocturnal intermittent peritoneal dialysis the abdomen is left dry during the day
C. Bicarbonate is the preferred buffer in the dialysate solutions
D. Pretreatment with quinine reduces the incidence of muscle cramps during dialysis
E. The most important cause of death in patients on haemodialysis is infection

Q 14. A 30-year-old man had a cadaveric renal transplant 5 months previously. He has suffered 2 episodes of rejection. The following are true except:

A. Hyperacute rejection is mediated by antibodies of the recipient towards the donor HLA class 1 antigens
B. Early rejection is an antibody mediated reaction
C. Native kidneys are likely to have been removed during renal transplantation
D. Okt3 is contraindicated in the treatment of acute rejection
E. Tacrolimus has a different mode of action from cyclosporine and so can be used if cyclosporine fails

A 12. C

A 13. E

A 14. A

Hypotension is a common complication during haemodialysis. It can be prevented by careful monitoring of the dry weight, avoiding antihypertensives on the day of dialysis, avoiding heavy meals before dialysis and can be managed by stopping ultrafiltration, infusing normal saline or salt free albumin, cooling the dialysate (Harrison).

Tenchkoff catheter is a cuffes catheter commonly used for peritoneal dialysis. In nocturnal intermittent dialysis 10 h of cycling is given in the night and the abdomen is left dry during the day. In continuous cyclic peritoneal dialysis 4–5 cycles are given in the night and the last exchange remains in the abdomen during the day. Bicarbonate is the preferred dialysate buffer and is used more commonly now than acetate. Increasing the sodium content of the dialysate and pretreatment with quinine reduces the incidence of muscle cramps during dialysis. Major cause of death in patients on dialysis is cardiovascular causes. Infection is also a major contributor.

Hyperacute rejection is mediated by antibodies to the donor HLA Type 1 antigens. This can be avoided by proper HLA matching. Early rejection is a T-cell mediated event. Chronic rejection produces nephrosclerosis. Calcineurin inhibitors like cyclosporine and tacrolimus can also produce early renal deterioration. Native kidneys are usually left in situ during transplantation. Okt3 is a monoclonal antibody directed against CD3 which forms a part of the T-cell receptor. It is very useful during the acute rejection episode. Cyclosporine has a similar mode of action as tacrolimus.

Immunosuppressive drug	Mechanism of action
Glucocorticoids	Blocks transcription of IL-1, 2, 3, 6, TNF-α
Cyclosporine	Trimolecular complex with cyclophillin and calcineurin block in IL-2 production
Tacrolimus	Same as cyclosporine
Azathioprine	Hepatic metabolites inhibit purine synthesis
Mycophenolate mofetil	Inhibits purine synthesis via inosine monophosphate dehydrogenase
Sirolimus	Blocks IL-2 receptor pathway

Glomerulonephritis, Etiology, Immunology, Prognosis and Treatment

Q 15. All of the following produce an acute nephritic syndrome with low levels of serum c3 except:

A. Lupus nephritis
B. Post streptococcal glomerulonephritis
C. Wegener's glomerulonephritis
D. Bacterial endocarditis
E. Cryoglobulinaemia

Q 16. P-ANCA is directed against which of the following antigens:

A. Myeloperoxidase
B. Proteinase-3
C. Neutrophil enolase
D. Elastase
E. Metalloproteinase

Q 17. A 50-year-old lady presents with 4 grams/24 hour proteinuria. Creatinine level is 120 μmol/l. A renal biopsy shows membranous glomerulopathy. The following are true of this condition:

A. Majority present with nephrotic syndrome
B. Complement levels are usually normal
C. HIV infection is a likely cause
D. Microscopic haematuria may be associated
E. Hepatitis B and C infection should be excluded

A 15. C

A 16. A

A 17. C

Acute glomerulonephritis with a reduced complement level in serum is usually associated with conditions like: poststreptococcal glomerulonephritis, lupus nephritis, MPGN, cryoglobulinaemia, bacterial endocarditis, shunt nephritis, etc. Wegener's, polyarteritis nodosa, etc produce usually an acute nephrotic or RPGN syndrome with pauciimmune deposits and normal serum complement. Antineutrophil cytoplasmic antibody can be of two types, cytoplasmic and nuclear. C-ANCA is usually directed against proteinase-3 antigen and commonly found in association with Wegener's. P-ANCA is usually associated with myeloperoxidase antigen and associated with PAN. These antibodies promote the activation and degranulation of cytokine primed neutrophils thereby contributing to the inflammatory process. Membranous glomerulonephritis is a common cause of nephrotic syndrome in adults. Light microscopy shows a thickening of glomerular basement membrane. It is associated with a lot of infective conditions like hepatitis, syphilis, leprosy, schistosomiasis, malaria, etc. HIV infection produces usually focal segmental glomerulosclerosis or MPGN. HIV can also infiltrate the kidney directly to produce renal failure. Microscopic haematuria is associated with membranous glomerulonephritis in about 50% of cases. Commonly causes nephrotic range proteinuria.

Some important associations
Minimal change disease
- Hodgkin's disease
- HIV infection
- Interferon alpha
- NSAIDs

Focal segmental glomerulosclerosis
- HIV
- Diabetes
- Charcot marietooth disease
- End stage of nephron loss from any cause
- Heroin addicts

MPGN/mesangiocapillary glomerulonephritis
- C3 nephritic factor, lipodystrophy, decreased c3 levels with normal c4 levels in type 2 MPGN

- Leukaemias, lymphomas, etc
- Sle, mctd, sjogrens, primary biliary cirrhosis
- Carcinoma: breast, colon, oesophagus, melanoma
- Gold, penicillamine, captopril
- Sarcoidosis, Crohn's, Guillain-Barre syndrome

IgA nephropathy
- Chronic liver disease
- Coeliac disease, Crohn's
- Henoch schonlein purpura
- Dermatitis herpetiformis

Membranous glomerulonephritis
- Hepatitis
- Syphilis
- Leprosy
- Schistosomiasis
- Malaria

Acute glomerulonephritis
Low complement
- Post streptococcal
- Lupus
- MPGN
- Cryoglobulinaemia
- Bacterial endocarditis
- Shunt nephritis

Aerial Complement
- Bacterial endocarditis
- Shunt nephritis

Acid Base Disorders

Q 18. The following bloods results are seen on an unwell patient:
pH 7.2, Na^+ 135 mmol/l, K^+ 5.5 mmol/l, HCO_3^- 12 mmol/l,
Cl^- 100 mmol/l. All the following are possible diagnoses except:

A. Diabetic ketoacidosis
B. Ureterosigmoidostomy
C. Lactic acidosis
D. Methanol poisoning
E. Chronic renal failure

Q 19. Which of the following is a factor in maintaining the reabsorption of bicarbonate in a patient with metabolic alkalosis?

A. Hypokalaemia
B. Low GFR
C. Low chloride
D. All of the above
E. None of the above

A 18. B

A 19. D

Normal anion gap is around 12–16 mmol. Anion gap is calculated by $Na^+ - [Cl^- + HCO_3^-]$. Urinary anion gap is measured by $[Na^+ + K^+]_{urine} - [Cl^-]_{urine}$. Uretero sigmoidostomy commonly causes a normal anion gap acidosis. Acidosis should be treated with alkali only if it is produced by conditions causing normal anion gap acidosis, or by a high anion gap acidosis due to a nonmetabolisable anion. Severe acidosis (pH <7.1), also should be treated with caution, the aim being to raise the pH >7.2 and to raise the bicarbonate to >15 mmol/l. Ethylene glycol/methanol intoxication should be treated with supportive measures, ethanol, fomepizol (new alcohol dehydrogenase inhibitor). Overenthusiastic treatment of DKA with alkali may lead to a worsening of the condition due to paradoxical acidosis, due to cardiovascular depression.

Hypokalaemia, low chloride, and decreased GFR all can hinder the renal compensation of excreting bicarbonate and lead to increased bicarbonate levels, thus maintaining the alkalosis. To compensate for alkalosis, more K^+ ions are lost, and so H^+ retained in the tubules of the kidney.

In acute respiratory acidosis the plasma bicarbonate raises by 1 mmol/l for every 10 mmHg raise in $PaCO_2$. In chronic respiratory acidosis, due to the renal compensation the bicarbonate level raises by 4 mmol/l for every 10 mmHg rise in $PaCO_2$.

Causes of high anion gap acidosis
- Lactic acidosis
- Diabetic keto acidosis
- Alcoholic keto acidosis
- Starvation ketosis
- Ethylene glycol toxicity
- Methanol toxicity
- Salicylates/paracetamol
- Renal failure (late stages)

Secondary Glomerulonephritis

Q 20. The following are features of diabetic nephropathy except:

    A. Glomerular hyperfiltration
    B. Microalbuminuria
    C. Diffuse glomerulosclerosis
    D. Nodular glomerulosclerosis
    E. Bilateral contracted kidneys

Q 21. A 30-year-old caucasian woman with system lupus erythematosus is found to have blood and protein in her urine. Renal biopsy suggests lupus nephritis. The following statements are true except:

    A. Serum complement level is decreased
    B. Anti DNA antibodies correlate the activity of lupus nephritis
    C. Drug induced lupus commonly presents with renal involvement
    D. Steroids and cyclophosphamide are the main stay of therapy
    E. WHO class 5 is associated with a better prognosis than class 4 lupus nephritis

A 20. E

A 21. C

Diabetic nephropathy starts with glomerular hyperfiltration and microalbuminuria 5–10 years after the onset. Microalbuminuria is defined as excretion of 30–300 mg/24 h of albumin spot urine alb/creatinine 30–300 mg/g. The pathologic features are GBM thickening, nodular glomerulosclerosis, mesangial expansion, diffuse glomerulosclerosis, etc. Immune deposits are not seen. ACE inhibitors are found to limit the progress to ESRD. Lupus nephritis is classified by WHO into 6 classes. Out of these class 4 is the most aggressive and 30% progress to ESRD. Class 2 and 5 may precede the systemic manifestations. Treatment is with steroids and cyclophosphamide. Double stranded DNA levels correlate with lupus nephritis. Drug induced lupus rarely presents with nephritis (anti-histone +).

Drugs and kidney
Minimal change disease
1. NSAIDs
2. IFN-α
3. Rifampicin
4. Ampicillin

Membranous nephritis
1. Penicillamine
2. Gold
3. Captopril
4. Trimethadione

Proliferative glomerulonephritis and RPGN
1. Allopurinol
2. Penicillin
3. Sulphonamides
4. Thiazides
5. Warfarin
6. Carbimazole
7. Amoxicillin

CRF and normal size kidneys
▪ Diabetes mellitus
▪ Adult polycystic kidney disease
▪ Amyloidosis

Types of lupus nephritis
1 – Normal renal biopsy
2 – Mesangial
3 – Focal segmental proliferative
4 – Diffuse proliferative
5 – Membranes
6 – End stage

Nephrolithiasis

Q 22. **A 40-year-old man presents with renal colic. A KUB X-ray shows no stone, but ultrasound suggests a 5 mm stone in the right renal pelvis. What is the composition of the stone likely to be?**

    A. Calcium oxalate
    B. Calcium phosphate
    C. Uric acid
    D. Cystine
    E. Hydroxyapatite

Q 23. **The following are true about renal stones except:**

    A. Struvite stones are formed by a complex of magnesium, ammonium and phosphate
    B. Thiazide diuretics are useful in preventing formation of calcium stones
    C. Low urinary citrate predisposes to renal stone formation
    D. Uric acid stones are predominantly formed when the urine is alkaline
    E. Cystinuria is always associated with dibasic aminoaciduria

A 22.   C

A 23.   D

Renal stones are radioopaque in 90% of cases, while gall stones are radiolucent in around 80% of cases. Cystine stones are radioopaque due to their sulphur content. Uric acid stones are radiolucent, but birefringent. Any renal stone less than 0.5cm usually pass through the ureter spontaneously. All stones are more frequent in men except struvite stones, which are more common in females. Thiazide diuretics reduce renal excretion of calcium and are useful in prevention of calcium stones. The hypokalaemia due to the diuresis should be treated as low potassium can reduce the urinary citrate and predispose to stone formation. Renal stones are common in distal renal tubular acidosis. Struvite stones are commonly associated with infections of the urinary tract and consist of ammonium, magnesium and phosphate. These stones and calcium phosphate stones precipitate in an alkaline urine. Uric acid stones and up to an extent cystine and calcium oxalate stones tends to precipitate more in acidic urine. Hemiacridine is a chemical that can dissolve struvite stones. Aceto hydroxamic acid is an inhibitor of urease and may help in preventing struvite stones. Cystinuria may or may not be associated with dibasic aminoaciduria.

Interesting points
Hyperoxaluria: can be hereditary or acquired. Hereditary is usually autosomal recessive trait.
Acquired:
1.   Bacterial overgrowth
2.   Jejunoileal bypass
3.   Chronic pancreatitis
4.   Ethylene glycol and methoxyflurane intoxication
Treatment: cholestyramine, calcium supplements, high fluid, pyridoxine.
Hypocitraturia: can be secondary to renal tubular acidosis, chronic diarrhoeal illness, hypokalaemia. Treatment is with alkali supplementation preferably potassium citrate.
Cystinuria: cystinuria usually due to a transport defect of dibasic aminoacids: COAL (cystine, ornithine, arginine, lysine). But may occur singly also.
Treatment: fluids, raising urinary pH, low salt diet, captopril.

Urinary Tract Infections

Q 24. Which of the following statements is true?

   A. Mid stream urinary culture with <1 lac colony count is significant and can be taken to denote infection usually
   B. P blood group negative individuals are more prone for pyelonephritis
   C. Emphysematous pyelonephritis are usually associated with diabetes mellitus
   D. All cases of asymptomatic bacteriuria should be treated
   E. One single episode of pyelonephritis in an adult male does not require urological investigation for a cause

Q 25. Which of the following conditions does not warrant treatment with antibiotics?

   A. Acute prostatitis
   B. Acute cystitis uncomplicated
   C. Acute pyelonephritis
   D. Prostatodynia
   E. Papillary necrosis

A 24. C

A 25. D

Colony count more than 1 lac/ml only is significant in a mid stream sample, while any bacteria colony in a suprapubic aspiration sample is considered significant. Catheterised samples with more than 1,000 colony count/ml is significant (Harrison). P blood group antigen acts as the receptor for certain bacterial species to gain entry into the urothelium and the incidence of pyelonephritis has been found to be less in patients with P antigen negative. Emphysematous pyelonephritis is associated usually with diabetes and is associated with formation of fermented gas in the renal tissue. Surgical resection is usually necessary. All cases of asymptomatic bacteriuria need not be treated and treatment may even lead to emergence of resistant strains. Only patients with neutropenia, complicated bacteriuria, renal transplants, pregnancy, etc need be treated. Acute uncomplicated cystitis is usually treated with quinolones or tmp-smz for 3 days. Acute pyelonephritis is treated with quinolones, cephalosporins, aztreonam, etc for 14 days. Prostatodynia is usually not associated with an infectious etiology and is not treated with antibiotics.

Neurology

Ptosis

Q 1. A 57-year-old man presents with a short history of unilateral ptosis. Which of the following is <u>not</u> part of the differential diagnosis?

A. Myasthenia gravis
B. A lesion of the third nerve nucleus
C. Horner's syndrome
D. Uncal herniation
E. Cavernous sinus thrombosis

Q 2. A 25-year-old woman is noted to have left-sided ptosis and miosis. Which of the following findings suggests an acquired, central lesion?

A. Pain in the axilla
B. Loss of sweating confined to the face
C. Hydroxyamphetamine 1% drops dilate the affected pupil
D. Heterochromia
E. Apparent enophthalmos

A 1. B

A 2. C

Ptosis is drooping of the eyelid. It is caused by weakness either of the smooth muscle innervating the eyelid (Müller's muscle) or of levator palpebrae superioris. The former is controlled by the sympathetic supply to the eye and is therefore impaired in Horner's syndrome. The latter is controlled by the third nerve. The **cause of levator palpebrae superioris weakness** depends on the level at which the III nerve is affected as follows:

Supranuclear:	large cortical infarct, demyelination, progressive supranuclear palsy
Nuclear:	brainstem infarct, demyelination, tumour
Nerve:	posterior communicating artery aneurysm, meningitis, uncal herniation, cavernous sinus thrombosis, tumour
NM Junction:	myasthenia gravis, Lambert-Eaton syndrome
Muscle:	myotonic dystrophy, oculopharyngeal muscular dystrophy, mitochondrial disorders

- Ptosis caused by muscle and neuromuscular junction disorders is commonly bilateral but may be unilateral, especially in myasthenia gravis.
- The third nerve nucleus is subdivided into distinct motor pools subserving individual extra-ocular muscles. The caudal nucleus, which controls levator palpebrae superioris, is a single midline structure and therefore isolated ptosis produced by any nuclear cause will always be bilateral.

Horner's syndrome consists of ipsilateral ptosis, miosis and anhydrosis. It is caused by interruption of the sympathetic supply to the eye. The pathway starts in the ipsilateral hypothalamus and has three neurones, which synapse first in the lateral grey of the spinal cord at T1 and second in the superior cervical sympathetic ganglion. Causes depend on the level of the lesion:

Brainstem:	tumour, demyelination, infarction
Cervical cord:	syringomyelia, tumour, demyelination
T1 root:	Pancoast syndrome, cervical ribs, trauma
Cervical sympathetic chain:	thyroid carcinoma, carotid body tumour, surgery
Internal carotid:	dissection

Pancoast syndrome is the triad of Horner's syndrome, wasting of the small muscles of the hand, and pain in the axilla, and results from damage to the T1 root. The commonest cause is an apical lung tumour; it occasionally also accompanies aneurysms of the subclavian artery.

In the absence of other signs, localisation may be aided by the pattern of loss of sweating and pharmacological tests. Loss of sweating in central lesions occurs over the ipsilateral head, arm and upper trunk, whereas it may be entirely absent in lesions distal to the superior sympathetic ganglion. Variable impairment in sweating occurs in lesions between T1 and the superior sympathetic ganglion. Pharmacological tests are performed by examining the pupillary response to instillation of pharmacological agents as eye drops. The responses and their interpretation are given below.

Agent	Normal pupil	Central Horner's	Peripheral Horner's
Cocaine 4%	Dilates	No effect	No effect
Adrenaline 1:1000	No effect	No effect	Dilates
1% hydroxyamphetamine	Dilates	Dilates	No effect

The action of cocaine on the normal pupil depends on its blockade of noradrenaline re-uptake: if the pathway is interrupted at any level no noradrenaline can be released and therefore blockade has no effect. In postganglionic lesions, degeneration of the terminal bulb sensitises the pupil to the action of 1:1000 adrenaline owing to receptor upregulation and the absence of amine oxidase at the nerve terminal. 1% hydroxyamphetamine stimulates the release of noradrenaline from the terminal bulb, it therefore has no effect in peripheral lesions where no noradrenaline is available for release.

Heterochromia refers to different pigmentation of the iris compared to the normal eye and is a feature of congenital Horner's syndrome. The affected eyeball often seems sunken (enophthalmos) owing to slight elevation of the lower eyelid.

Neurology

Ptosis

Chorea

Q 3. A 45-year-old woman is found to have flitting, jerky, purposeless movements of her upper limbs. Which of the following is least likely to be relevant to the diagnosis?

A. Past exposure to carbon monoxide
B. Taking the oral contraceptive pill
C. Evidence of recent streptococcal infection
D. Vitamin A supplements
E. A history of deep venous thrombosis

Q 4. A 20-year-old man is admitted with acute psychosis. He is noted to have dysarthria, dystonic posturing of his left hand, and generalised rigidity. Investigations reveal absent caeruloplasmin. Which of the following additional features is unlikely?

A. Renal tubular acidosis
B. Reduced copper levels in bile
C. Reticulocytosis
D. Glucose intolerance
E. Cystic changes within the brainstem

A 3. D

A 4. D

Rapid, jerky, purposeless movements, which often flit from one part of the body to another, are characteristic of chorea. When associated with slower, sinuous, writhing movements (athetosis) it is termed choreoathetosis. Chorea results from damage to the basal ganglia, particularly caudate nucleus and putamen, and is associated with hyperfunction of dopaminergic pathways and hypofunction of GABA-ergic and cholinergic pathways in the striatum. Violent, large amplitude chorea is termed ballism, this may be uni- or bilateral and is most commonly caused by ischaemic damage to the contralateral subthalamic nucleus.

Chorea is almost always symptomatic of an underlying disease. Other types of dyskinesia frequently accompany it.

Causes

Neurodegenerative:	Huntington's disease
	Benign hereditary chorea
	Dentatorubropallidoluysian atrophy
Inherited metabolic:	Wilson's disease
	Lesch-Nyhan disease
	Neuroacanthosis
Hypoxic/ischaemic:	Stroke
	Hypotension
	Vasculitis
	Sickle cell disease
	Polycythaemia
Toxic:	Copper
	Mercury
Drug induced:	Oral contraceptive pill
	L-Dopa
	Neuroleptics
	Anticholinergics
	Cocaine
	Amphetamines
Infection:	Sydenham's chorea
	Meningitis
	Viral encephalitis
	Mycoplasma pneumoniae
	Legionella
	Toxoplasmosis
	Creutzfeld-Jacob disease
Autoimmune:	SLE
	Primary anti-phospholipid syndrome
	Vasculitis
	Behcet's
	Hashimoto's thyroiditis (unrelated to hyperthyroidism)
Endocrine:	Thyrotoxicosis
	Chorea gravidarum
	Addison's disease
Metabolic:	Hypocalcaemia
	Hypomagnesaemia
	Hyper/hypoglycaemia
	Hyper/hyponatraemia

Carbon monoxide binds to haemoglobin and cytochromes thereby leading to cellular hypoxia and brain damage. Severe poisoning is associated with diffuse neuronal loss in the cerebral cortex, basal ganglia, and limbic system and manifests as multifocal neurological abnormalities including cognitive dysfunction and extrapyramidal features including, rarely, chorea. Survivors of severe poisoning may develop a delayed leukoencephalopathy weeks after the primary insult.

Chorea is one of the major criteria for the diagnosis of rheumatic fever, which occurs following Group A streptococcal pharyngitis. A history of deep venous thrombosis may suggest the anti-phospholipid syndrome, either in isolation, or as part of systemic lupus erythematosus. Vitamin A excess does not cause chorea but can be associated with a syndrome resembling idiopathic intracranial hypertension.

Wilson's disease is an autosomal recessive disorder characterised by accumulation of copper in the body (principally liver, brain and kidneys), deficient caeruloplasmin synthesis, and reduced biliary copper excretion. The affected gene (*WND*) is located on chromosome 13 and codes for an ATPase which is implicated in the excretion of copper in bile. The prevalence is 1 per 30,000. The majority of patients present before middle age and the initial presentation is neurological in 40%.

The neurological picture is dominated by extrapyramidal features, particularly facial and bulbar dystonia (leading to dysarthria, dysphagia and drooling of saliva), limb dystonias, rigidity, and tremor. Occasionally incoordination, ataxia, and psychiatric disturbance are early features. Almost all patients in whom neurological features are present have Kayser-Fleischer rings. These are caused by deposition of copper in Descemet's membrane, and are sometimes seen in other conditions associated with impaired copper elimination such as primary biliary cirrhosis. The non-neurological features include a wide spectrum of liver abnormalities, renal disease (Fanconi's syndrome, proximal or distal renal tubular acidosis, osteomalacia), cataracts, Coombs-negative haemolytic anaemia, osteoarthritis and, rarely, cardiac hypertrophy.

Investigation findings are reduced or absent serum caeruloplasmin (95% of patients), elevated 24 h urinary copper excretion, and increased hepatic copper load on liver biopsy. First line treatment remains the copper chelating agent D-penicillamine; triethylene tetramine and ammonium thiomolybdate are alternatives.

Complications of penicillamine
- Hypersensitivity reactions
- Neutropenia
- Thrombocytopenia
- Skin rashes
- Nephrotic syndrome
- Myasthenia gravis
- Goodpasture's syndrome
- Systemic lupus erythematosus

Facial Nerve

Q 5. Following a road traffic accident, a young biker suffers traumatic damage to the facial nerve. Which of the following statements is not correct?

    A. Transection proximal to the origin of the greater petrosal nerve would result in loss of taste from the palate
    B. Transection can produce loss of sensation in the ear canal
    C. Unilateral damage to the facial nerve can produce bilateral weakness of the frontalis muscle
    D. Lesion above the stylomastoid foramen would affect the nerve to stapedius
    E. Taste fibres from the anterior two thirds of the tongue are carried in the lingual nerve and chorda tympani

Q 6. A 30-year-old woman is noted to have bilateral facial weakness and a bulbar palsy. Which of the following diagnoses is hardest to reconcile with the clinical picture?

    A. Multiple sclerosis
    B. Syringomyelia
    C. Guillain-Barre syndrome
    D. Sarcoidosis
    E. Polio

A 5. C

A 6. B

The facial nerve carries motor, sensory and parasympathetic fibres.

Motor fibres originate in the facial motor nucleus in the ventrolateral pons, sweep dorsomedially around the sixth nerve nucleus, emerge from the lateral border of the pons at the cerebellopontine angle, enter the petrous bone though the internal auditory meatus, course through the facial canal, unite with the fibres of the intermediate nerve at the geniculate ganglion, and exit from the stylomastoid foramen to innervate the stylohyoid muscle, posterior belly of digastric and finally all the muscles of facial expression excluding levator palpebrae superioris. A small branch to the stapedius muscle leaves the facial canal 6 mm proximal to the stylomastoid foramen.

Sensory fibres have their cell bodies in the geniculate ganglion and are of two types: cutaneous nerve fibres subserving a small area of skin in the external auditory meatus and behind the ear, and special visceral afferent fibres conveying taste sensation from the anterior 2/3rd of the tongue and part of the palate. The former join the nerve at the stylomastoid foramen and travel in the intermediate nerve to terminate in the spinal trigeminal tract. The latter follow two pathways. The fibres from the anterior 2/3rd of the tongue travel via the lingual nerve then corda tympani and intermediate nerve, finally terminating in the nucleus solitarius in the medulla. The fibres from the palate travel in the greater petrosal nerve and join the first pathway at the geniculate ganglion.

Preganglionic parasympathetic originate from the superior salivary nucleus, travel in the intermediate nerve and divide at the geniculate ganglion to supply the pterygopalatine ganglion via the superficial petrosal nerve, and the submandibular ganglion via the chorda tympani. Postganglionic fibres from the pterygopalatine ganglion innervate the lacrimal gland and mucosa of the mouth and nose, and those from the submandibular ganglion innervate the submandibular and sublingual salivary glands. Note that the parasympathetic supply to the parotid gland is relayed via the glossopharyngeal and not the facial nerve.

The facial nerve nuclei are under complex supranuclear control. The cells responsible for driving the upper facial muscles receive inputs from both hemispheres. In addition, there are inputs from fibres originating from subcortical structures. The clinical consequences of this are that in a unilateral upper motor neurone lesion the upper facial muscles will be spared, and the weakness will be less apparent if the facial movement is driven by emotion rather than volition.

Multiple sclerosis may give rise to bilateral facial nerve palsies through damage either to descending corticobulbar fibres, or to the facial nerve nuclei and their fascicles in the pons. Syringomyelia will not unless the syrinx has extended rostrally and has given rise to syringobulbia. Facial nerve palsy in Guillain-Barre syndrome may be uni- or bilateral. Sarcoidosis may produce a chronic basal meningitis (in which case other cranial nerve palsies may be present); the facial nerves may also be involved in their extracranial course if the parotid glands are affected. Acute polio more commonly damages the motor neurones in the lower cranial nuclei, but the facial may occasionally be involved.

Causes of bilateral VIIth nerve palsy

Upper motor neurone/nuclear	Lower motor neurone
Motor neurone disease	Sarcoid
Diffuse cerebrovascular disease	Polio
Pontine infarct	Guillain-Barre syndrome
Multiple sclerosis	Vasculitis
	Lyme disease
	HIV
	Melkersson's syndrome

Meningitis and Encephalitis

Q 7. **Which of the following statements concerning meningitis is incorrect?**

A. Almost all cases of amoebic meningitis occur in the immunosuppressed

B. Cefotaxime does not adequately treat listeria meningitis

C. Mumps meningitis may be associated with low glucose levels in the CSF

D. Treatment with dexamethasone may be indicated

E. Hydrocephalus occurs in 5% of cases of pyogenic meningitis

Q 8. **Which of the following statements is correct?**

A. Progressive multifocal leukoencephalopathy is caused by BK virus

B. The incidence of post-infectious measles encephalitis is 1 in 1,000 cases

C. Mucormycosis is usually adequately treated pharmacologically

D. Cystercercosis is associated with seizures in a minority of cases

E. Whipple's disease very rarely presents with isolated neurological features

$\boxed{A}$ 7. A

$\boxed{A}$ 8. B

Mumps meningitis is possibly the only viral cause of meningitis associated with a low glucose level in the CSF. In cases of bacterial meningitis dexamethasone therapy reduces the incidence of neurological sequelae in children; whether there is any benefit in adults is matter of dispute. Hydrocephalus resulting from meningeal adhesions occurs in about 5% of cases of bacterial meningitis and may present years after the event.

Amoebic meningitis is usually caused by infection with either of two types of free-living amoebae. *Naegleria fowleri* is found in warm, stagnant fresh-water and infects immunocompetent people probably by entering the brain via the cribriform plate when contaminated water comes into contact with the nasal mucosa during swimming. It causes an acute purulent meningoencephalitis that is difficult to distinguish from bacterial infection unless amoebae are looked for in the cerebrospinal fluid using phase-contrast microscopy. A history of exposure to water is often the only clue. Treatment is with amphotericin B; the prognosis is usually poor. *Acanthamoeba* infection causes a focal granulomatous meningoencephalitis in immunocompromised individuals usually from haematogenous spread from primary infection in the eye, sinuses, middle ear, lung, or gastric wall. *Unlike infection* with *Naegleria fowleri* trophozoites are usually not seen in the CSF and diagnosis is usually made histologically.

Listeria monocytogenes may cause meningitis in normal people but is more common in pregnant women, the elderly, and the immunosuppressed. A fifth of all cases are attributable to eating contaminated foods such as unpasteurised cheese, vegetables, and undercooked meat. The clinical and laboratory features resemble bacterial infection with a conventional organism although the onset may be more protracted and brainstem signs are more common. Treatment is with amoxicillin and gentamicin; the mortality is usually high. It is often forgotten that the organism is relatively resistant to most cephalosporins.

Progressive multifocal leukoencephalopathy is an invariably fatal CNS infection caused by the JC virus. This papovavirus is an almost ubiquitous finding in normal renal tissue where it causes a persistent latent infection without any accompanying symptoms. Reactivation occurs exclusively in the immunosuppressed leading to lytic infection of oligodendrocytes with resultant areas of demyelination throughout the brain. The presentation depends on the area of brain affected. Diagnosis relies on the characteristic appearance on MRI and detection of virus in the CSF by PCR. No satisfactory treatment exists, although there is anecdotal evidence that survival in AIDS patients may be prolonged by successful anti-retroviral therapy.

Measles causes three distinct types of encephalitis: postinfectious encephalitis, measles inclusion body encephalitis and subacute sclerosing panencephalitis. The first is by far the commonest, occurring in 1:1000 cases of measles, principally in patients over the age of 2. The clinical features are of a rapidly progressive encephalopathy with confusion, convulsions, paresis, ataxia and myoclonus, occurring within a week of the onset of the rash. Virus is rarely isolated from brain and it appears most of the damage is immunologically mediated. The incidence of long term neurological sequelae is high. Subacute inclusion body encephalitis occurs in the immunosuppressed and develops insidiously several months after the attack of measles. Inclusion bodies signifying viral replication are seen, and viral antigens may be isolated from brain. It is invariably fatal. Subacute sclerosing panencephalitis is a rare complication of measles (5 per million cases), which develops several years after the primary illness. The onset is insidious with psychological and cognitive changes, ataxia, clumsiness and seizures. Later, myoclonus, pyramidal and extrapyramidal signs appear, and the disease inexorably progresses to a vegetative state and death in the vast majority.

The rate of decline varies from weeks to several months. There is no treatment and the only protection is immunisation.

Mucormycosis is infection caused by members of the Mucoraceae family. The majority of cases occur in diabetic patients who are acidotic for some reason, the rest occur in patients who are immunosuppressed or debilitated. The infection is usually initiated in the facial sinuses and spreads to the brain contiguously or haematogenously. Arterial thrombosis, infarction, and aneurysm formation, occur with associated focal neurological signs. Embolisation may lead to abscesses at distant sites. Aggressive treatment of the predisposing condition, surgical debridement, and anti-fungal agents may help, but the prognosis is usually poor.

Cystercercosis is caused by infection with the pork tapeworm *Taenia solium*. It is widespread in the developing world and it is the commonest cause of epilepsy worldwide. Man (the definitive host) acquires the worm by eating pork from infected pigs (the intermediate host). The worms reside in the human intestine and produce large numbers of eggs, which are subsequently ingested by pigs fed contaminated food, thus completing the cycle. If man ingests the eggs through faeco-oral contamination he can become the intermediate host; the eggs hatch in the gastrointestinal tract and are distributed via the bloodstream to many tissues, including muscle and brain. Neurological symptoms occur when cerebral cysts cause seizures, hydrocephalus or cranial nerve palsies. If the lesion load is large, inadvertent treatment (e.g. for infection with another parasite) with anti-parasitic agents to which the cystercerca are susceptible can cause severe brain oedema owing to a brisk inflammatory response to the dying organisms. Treatment is surgery for space-occupying lesions and hydrocephalus, and anti-epileptic drugs for seizures. Where specific treatment is indicated praziquantel or albendazole may be used to eliminate the cysts.

Whipple's disease a systemic illness caused by infection with the bacillus *Tropheryma whippelii*. Neurological symptoms occur in a substantial proportion of patients and in 5% may be the only manifestation of the disease. The neurological features are varied and include dementia, tremor, movement abnormalities, seizures, ophthalmoplegia and ataxia. A specific type of movement disorder involving eye movements, oculomasticatory myorhythmia, is diagnostic. The diagnosis is confirmed by finding *T. whippelii* DNA by PCR of affected tissue. Treatment is with a long course of parenteral cephalosporin or combination of penicillin and streptomycin. Relapse is common.

Papilloedema

Q 9. A 57-year-old homeless man presents with a complaint of headache. On examination he is obese and has bilateral papilloedema. Which of the following is not part of the differential diagnosis?

A. Methanol poisoning
B. Benign intracranial hypertension
C. Normal pressure hydrocephalus
D. Frontal meningioma
E. Severe hypercapnoea

Q 10. A 36-year-old woman presents with a 2-month history of constant, daily headache and transient blurring of vision. The only positive findings on examination are obesity and bilateral papilloedema. CT head is normal. Which of the following is least likely to be relevant to the final diagnosis?

A. History of acne
B. History of deep venous thrombosis
C. Recent treatment with corticosteroids
D. Development of a unilateral sixth nerve palsy
E. Mild hyponatraemia

A 9. C

A 10. D

Papilloedema is swelling of the optic disc. It occurs either from raised intracranial pressure or focal damage to the optic bulb caused by acute inflammation, infection, or ischaemia. Where the cause is raised intracranial pressure the patient may report transient diminution in visual acuity associated with manoeuvres that raise the pressure further such as coughing or Valsalva; this phenomenon is termed obscuration. The earliest funduscopic sign of papilloedema is loss of venous pulsation; however this is seen in 20% of normal people.

Causes

Space-occupying lesions
- Tumour
- Abscess
- Granulomas
- Cysts
- Intracerebral haemorrhage

Intracranial infection
- Meningitis
- Encephalitis

Obstructed venous outflow
- Venous sinus thrombosis
- Superior vena cava thrombosis
- A-V malformation
- Central retinal vein thrombosis

Obstructive hydrocephalus

'Benign' intracranial hypertension
- Idiopathic
- Hypervitaminosis A
- Retinoid derivatives
- Tetracyclines
- Steroids

Thyrotoxicosis

Hypoparathyroidism

Severe anaemia

Optic neuritis
- Ischaemic (e.g. DM, vasculitis, hyperviscosity)
- Inflammatory (e.g. demyelination, sarcoidosis)
- Toxic (e.g. methanol, heavy metals)
- Drugs (e.g. ethambutol, chloroquine)

Optic nerve compression

Malignant hypertension

Hypercapnoea

Guillain-Barré syndrome

Head injury

Benign (idiopathic) intracranial hypertension is a fairly common condition characterised by persistent elevated intracranial pressure in the absence of any abnormality on imaging. The pathological process is uncertain but may involve increased CSF production or impaired reabsorption. It usually occurs in obese women, with a peak incidence in middle age. There are associations with pregnancy, and treatment with the oral contraceptive pill, steroids, tetracyclines, and Vitamin A and its derivatives. Patients complain of headache, obscurations, and occasionally diplopia if a sixth nerve palsy resulting from the raised intracranial pressure is present. Other cranial nerve palsies do not occur. Fundoscopy shows papilloedema and the resulting damage to the optic nerve is the main hazard of the condition. Treatment consists of removing precipitants, weight loss, CSF drainage by repeated lumbar puncture, and acetazolamide. In severe cases high dose dexamethasone may be used, and if vision is threatened optic nerve sheath fenestration may be performed to relieve pressure on the optic nerve.

Cerebral venous sinus thrombosis may occasionally mimic BIH exactly. Diagnosis is made either by magnetic resonance venography or conventional angiography. Suspicions should be raised if there is any evidence of a prothrombotic tendency (such as a past history of DVT) or there are no risk factors for the idiopathic condition; some centres perform non-invasive imaging on all patients.

When considering conditions that may be associated with pregnancy it is important to remember that some women may be unaware that they are pregnant. Mild hyponatraemia, anaemia, and hypoalbuminaemia; and mildly raised alkaline phosphatase may be the only clues available to the physician.

Tremor

Q 11. A 63-year-old man presents with a complaint of hand tremor. On examination he has mild postural instability, increased rigidity in both upper limbs, and hand tremor on the left. Power is normal and there are no sensory signs. Which of the following would not make a diagnosis of Parkinson's disease less likely?

A. Impaired downgaze
B. Postural hypotension
C. Poor response to levodopa
D. Mild cognitive slowing
E. Upper limb hypermetria

Q 12. A 50-year-old man presents with hand tremor. On examination, he has fine, bilateral, postural hand tremor. There are no other abnormalities. Which of the following would be unexpected?

A. Evidence of recessive inheritance
B. Presence of titubation
C. Improvement with alcohol
D. Presence of mild intention tremor
E. Involvement of the tongue

A 11. D

A 12. A

Parkinson's disease is the commonest cause of parkinsonism. The prevalence is 100–250 per 100,000 and the age of onset is commonly after 50. The aetiology is unclear although environmental toxins have been implicated. It is characterised clinically by bradykinesia, rigidity, tremor and postural instability; and pathologically by loss of dopaminergic neurones in the substantia nigra and the presence of Lewy bodies in the brain. It is distinguished from other forms of parkinsonism on the basis of fairly asymmetrical onset, lack of atypical features (such as absent tremor, cerebellar or pyramidal signs, ophthalmoplegia, autonomic features or rapid progression) and good response to treatment with levodopa. Cognitive impairment is seen in about a third, and tends to follow a subcortical pattern with cognitive slowing, depression and memory impairment. Pharmacological treatment is with anticholinergic drugs, levodopa, dopamine agonists, selegeline and occasionally amantadine. Stereotactic thalamotomy or implantation of thalamic stimulators is used in patients resistant to medical treatment.

Causes of parkinsonism
Parkinson's disease
Other degenerative conditions
- Progressive supranuclear palsy
- Multisystem atrophy
- Parkinson-dementia-amyotrophic lateral sclerosis complex
- Huntington's disease (Westphal variant)
- Corticobasal degeneration
- Hallervorden-Spatz disease
- Neuroacanthocytosis

Drugs
- Dopamine antagonists
- Lithium
- SSRIs

Toxins
- Carbon monoxide
- Manganese
- Mercury
- MPTP

Vascular

Post-encephalitic

Metabolic
- Wilson's
- Storage diseases

Head injury

Essential tremor may be sporadic but has autosomal dominant inheritance in the majority. It causes predominantly postural tremor of at a rate of 4–12 Hz which affects initially the upper limbs but may subsequently spread to involve the legs, head (titubation), tongue and voice. There may be a mild intention component, and in about half mild ataxia of gait is seen. The tremor characteristically shows a temporary response to alcohol and this feature together with the absence of rigidity and bradykinesia allow it to be differentiated from parkinsonism. Treatment with propranolol is usually effective; severe cases may require bilateral thalamotomy or better still bilateral thalamic stimulation.

Spinal Cord Lesions

Q 13. **A 55-year-old man presents with sudden onset of paraplegia. Which of the following statements is correct?**

    A. Lack of spasticity within hours of the event suggests a peripheral cause

    B. The lesion must be in the spinal cord

    C. The patient should be treated with anti-platelet agents if MRI of the spine is normal

    D. A sensory level accurately localises the lesion

    E. The finding of dissociated sensory loss is helpful clinically

Q 14. **A 45-year-old woman is found to have a central cord lesion at C6. Which of the following cannot be explained by her lesion?**

    A. Bilateral Horner's syndrome

    B. Wasting of deltoid

    C. Sensory loss over the lateral forearm

    D. Loss of supinator jerk

    E. Spastic paraparesis

A 13. E

A 14. B

Although spastic paraparesis is most commonly caused by myelopathy, it may be caused by damage to any part of the corticospinal tract. The areas of the motor cortex that subserve leg function map close to the midline; therefore a lesion in the anterior midline such as a falx meningioma may give rise to spastic paraparesis owing to compression of the corticospinal fibres.

Acute transection of the cord leads to complete flaccid paralysis and sensory loss below the level of the lesion; signs of spasticity develop hours to days later. Myelopathy of sudden onset is most commonly caused by a vascular insult; in such cases there is often sparing of the sensory modalities subserved by the dorsal columns because the posterior parts of the cord have a separate blood supply. When this occurs in the thoracic region occlusion of the anterior spinal artery due to aortic dissection needs to be considered especially in the presence of back pain, although embolisation or thrombosis within the artery are more common causes. Clearly an aortic aneurysm will not be revealed by magnetic resonance imaging of the spinal cord alone.

Because sensory fibres entering the cord are topographically arranged, a spinal cord lesion may cause a sensory level anywhere below the level of the lesion depending on which fibres are affected. Therefore a sensory level is only a reliable guide to the lowest possible level of the lesion. Recovery following a vascular insult to the spinal cord is generally poor.

Causes of myelopathy

Compressive
- Tumour
  - Intrinsic
  - Bone
  - Metastases
  - Myeloma
- Prolapsed disc
- Vertebral abscess
- Haematoma
- Fracture

Vascular
- Anterior spinal artery occlusion
- Thromboembolism
- Venous thrombosis
- Caisson's disease
- Aortic dissection
- Vasculitis
- Fibrocartilagenous embolism

Inflammatory
- Multiple sclerosis
- Devic's syndrome
- Sarcoid
- Behcet's
- Post-infectious

Infective
- Spinal cord abscess
- Myelitis
  - Viral
  - Lyme
  - Atypicals
- Syphilis
- Brucella
- Schistosomiasis

The features of a **central cord lesion** will depend on its location, its cross-sectional diameter, and its extent along the craniocaudal axis. An early sign is usually impairment in temperature and pain sensation at the level of the lesion, either uni- or bilaterally, because fibres subserving these modalities cross near the midline within a few segments of entering the cord in order to ascend in the spinothalamic tract on the contralateral side. If the lesion is above T1 a Horner's syndrome may be produced because sympathetic fibres travel close to the midline as they descend in the spinal cord. As the lesion expands in diameter the anterior horn cells will be affected leading to weakness and wasting at the level of the lesion. On further expansion the corticospinal, spinothalamic tracts, and lastly dorsal column tracts will be affected leading to signs below the level of the lesion. In the case described in the question wasting of deltoid will not occur because its root value (C5) is above the level of the lesion.

Syringomyelia is the commonest central cord syndrome. It is associated with the formation and progressive expansion of a fluid-filled cavity in the centre of the cord, most commonly in the cervical and upper thoracic region. The mechanism of syrinx formation is unclear but seems to be associated with abnormalities at the craniocervical junction, particularly the Chiari malformation (congenital prolapse of the cerebellar tonsils through the foramen magnum). Other causes include trauma, basal arachnoiditis, and spinal tumours. The clinical picture is that of a gradually progressive central cord lesion as described above. In the sensory domain, either uni- or bilateral pain and temperature loss in the lower cervical segments is the earliest sign. As the lesion expands along the craniocaudal axis this dissociated sensory loss spreads rostrally to encroach onto the face in a 'cape' distribution and caudally to produce a suspended sensory level on the thorax. Later the spinothalamic tracts and dorsal columns below the level of the lesion are affected. In the motor domain, the earliest sign is weakness and wasting of the hand and forearm muscles which later spreads to involve muscles subserved by higher cervical segments. This is followed by pyramidal weakness below the level of the lesion occurs owing to compression of the corticospinal tract. Autonomic disturbance occurs owing to interruption of sympathetic pathways travelling medially in the cord which leads to uni- or bilateral Horner's syndrome and, together with anaesthesia, this contributes to trophic changes in the upper limbs. The diagnosis is confirmed on magnetic resonance imaging. Progression is usually slow and treatment conservative; surgery may be considered, especially if the cause is a tumour or the Chiari malformation.

Narcolepsy and Epilepsy

Q 15. A 23-year-old man presents with brief episodes of collapse without loss of consciousness. On close questioning he admits to excessive sleepiness during the day and vivid hallucinations on waking. Which of the following features is unlikely to be associated?

A. Mild hypercapnoea
B. Response to treatment with clomipramine
C. Abnormal periods of early onset REM sleep
D. Distinct HLA haplotype
E. Sleep paralysis

Q 16. An 18-year-old girl presents with a suspected seizure. Which of the following features suggests generalised tonic/clonic seizures rather than pseudoseizures?

A. Absence of pupillary dilatation
B. Asynchronous movements
C. Pelvic thrusting
D. Gaze aversion
E. Stereotyped attacks

A 15. A

Narcolepsy is a disorder of sleep characterised by excessive daytime somnolence, cataplexy, and a range of sleep-related phenomena. It has an equal sex distribution and shows strong linkage with certain HLA haplotypes, especially DQB1-0602. The aetiology remains uncertain although a disturbance of hypothalamic signalling involving deficiency of the novel neuropeptide hypocretin has been implicated.

   Cataplexy is sudden loss of muscle tone lasting seconds to minutes that is triggered by strong emotion or surprise, and is present in the vast majority of narcoleptics. The sleep phenomena include vivid hallucinations on going to (hypnagogic) or waking from (hypnapompic) sleep, and sleep paralysis, which refers to a short-lived inability to move experienced on waking. There are usually no abnormalities on examination. Early onset REM sleep is characteristic of the disorder and is demonstrated on sleep studies. Treatment with clomipramine usually abolishes cataplexy, the somnolence is harder to treat although a variety of CNS stimulants have been used.

A 16. E

The distinction between real generalised seizures and pseudoseizures is often difficult to make, especially in patients who have both. The most helpful clinical features pointing to pseudoseizures are any evidence of voluntary activity during the episode (e.g. resistance to eye opening and passive limb movements, gaze aversion, prevention of patient's own hand falling on face), and the absence of pupillary dilatation which is said to be invariable in generalised seizures. Complex movements such as flailing of the limbs, rolling of the body or pelvic thrusting are rare in generalised seizures. The presence of tongue biting and incontinence may also be helpful. The absence of EEG abnormalities during an episode is very strong evidence against true seizures.

Muscle and Neuromuscular Junction Disease

Q 17. Which of the following statements concerning muscle disease is correct?

    A. Thyrotoxic myopathy is usually associated with raised creatinine kinase

    B. Hypothyroidism is a feature of myotonic dystrophy

    C. Inclusion body myositis responds to steroids

    D. Oculopharyngeal muscular dystrophy is associated with trinucleotide repeat expansions

    E. Duchenne muscular dystrophy is not associated with reduced IQ

Q 18. A 52-year-old man presents with indolent onset of bilateral ptosis which is worse at the end of the day. He also complains of intermittent diplopia, particularly on downgaze. On examination he has bilateral ptosis, impaired abduction and depression of the left eye, and mildly reduced abduction of the right eye. There is mild, symmetrical, weakness of both arms proximally. The rest of the examination is normal. Which of the following features is least likely to be relevant?

    A. Recent treatment with penicillamine

    B. Hyponatraemia

    C. Dry mouth

    D. History of hypothyroidism

    E. Improvement with azathioprine

A 17. D

A 18. A

Thyrotoxic myopathy occurs in about a third of thyrotoxic patients. It features predominantly shoulder girdle weakness with mild wasting and occasional fasciculations which are related to motor unit instability resulting from the thyrotoxic state rather than denervation. Typically the CK is normal. The condition remits on successful treatment of the endocrine disorder. Hypothyroidism also causes muscle weakness but it is much milder. A condition simulating hypokalaemic periodic paralysis may be seen in patients with thyrotoxicosis (especially Orientals), and when the thyrotoxicosis is of autoimmune origin, other organ-specific autoimmune diseases such as myasthenia gravis.

Myotonic dystrophy is the commonest inherited myopathy in adults with an incidence of 10 per 100,000. The genetic basis is expansion a CTG repeat and it therefore shows anticipation. The adult form presents in late adolescence or early adulthood. Skeletal muscle features include ptosis, facial wasting, and distal limb weakness with delayed muscle relaxation following contraction or percussion (myotonia). Respiratory muscle weakness occurs late. There are many manifestations of the illness which are unrelated to its effect on skeletal muscle:

Cataracts

Cardiac muscle:	arrhythmias
	cardiomyopathy
Smooth muscle:	dysphagia
	constipation
	incontinence
CNS:	low IQ
	daytime somnolence
Endocrine:	testicular atrophy
	reduced fertility
	male pattern baldness
	glucose intolerance

Inclusion body myositis is chronic myopathy most commonly affecting elderly males. It presents with proximal and distal weakness, and wasting characteristically affecting the finger flexors and quadriceps. Dysphagia occurs late. There are no extramuscular features. Creatinine kinase is elevated and electromyographic features resemble those seen in polymyositis. Biopsy shows characteristic 15 nm intracellular inclusions. Treatment with immunosuppression is largely ineffective.

Oculopharyngeal muscular dystrophy has autosomal dominant inheritance and is associated with trinucleotide repeat expansions. It presents with ptosis and mild external ophthalmoplegia after the age of 50 followed by dysphagia months to years later and finally (predominantly upper) limb girdle weakness. Management is symptomatic.

Conditions associated with trinucleotide repeat expansions
- Huntington's disease
- Myotonic dystrophy
- Fragile X
- X-linked bulbospinal neuronopathy
- Spinocerebellar ataxia
- Dentatorubropallidoluysian atrophy

Duchenne muscular dystrophy is caused by mutations in the dystrophin gene and has X-linked recessive inheritance. Girls with Turner's syndrome may be affected. The incidence is 30 per 100,000 males of which a third a new mutations. Clinically, progressive lower then upper limb weakness develops in the first year of life. Hypertrophy is most obvious in calves, quadriceps and masseters. Scoliosis develops as a result of weakness of axial musculature and together with respiratory muscle weakness leads to hypoventilation which may progress to respiratory failure. Cardiac involvement is universal but not commonly symptomatic; a small proportion develop heart failure. Most patients are mildly cognitively impaired with an average IQ of 80. Diagnosis is based on clinical features, raised CK, absence or deficiency of dystrophin on biopsy, and demonstration of the gene defect. Treatment is physiotherapy, prevention of contractures, non-invasive ventilation for respiratory failure, genetic counselling and psychological support.

    Myasthenia gravis is the commonest neuromuscular disorder with a prevalence of 5–10 per 100,000. Amongst younger patients it is commoner in women. In cases of generalised myasthenia antibodies to acetylcholine receptors are seen in 80%, this falls to 50% in cases of pure ophthalmoplegia. It is associated with rheumatoid arthritis, systemic lupus erythematosus, other organ-specific autoimmune disorders, and penicillamine treatment. Clinically, any muscle may be affected but ptosis, ophthalmoplegia and dysphagia are most common. Proximal weakness exceeds distal. Weakness tends to worsen during the day and increased fatiguability is characteristic. Emotion, infection and heat may exacerbate weakness.

    Diagnosis is by antiacetylcholine receptor antibodies, tensilon test, and EMG which shows a decremental response of the compound muscle action potential to repetitive nerve stimulation. A thymoma is present in about 10% of cases and should be removed although this does not usually improve the myasthenia. Symptomatic benefit is produced by oral anticholinesterases such as pyridostigmine. Specific treatment is with oral steroids (which may transiently worsen symptoms); azathioprine frequently needs to be added as a steroid-sparing agent. Plasma exchange can be used in rapidly worsening symptoms or if the disease is refractory to immunosuppressant treatment. A third of young patients with generalised myasthenia in whom the thymus is hyperplastic will benefit from thymectomy. Severe weakness associated with respiratory failure is termed myasthenic crisis; this may be confused with cholinergic crisis and should be managed by intubation and ventilation, withdrawal of anticholinesterase treatment, and plasma exchange or intravenous immunoglobulin.

    Myasthenia gravis is sometimes hard to distinguish from the **Lambert-Eaton Myasthenic Syndrome (LEMS)**, a disorder of the neuromuscular junction caused by antibodies to presynaptic voltage-gated calcium channels. It is frequently associated with malignancy, particularly small cell lung cancer, in which case it may be accompanied by other paraneoplastic syndromes such as SIADH. The clinical features are similar to myasthenia but the weakness usually affects the limbs proximally, and involvement of the ocular and pharyngeal musculature is less common. In addition, autonomic features such as dry mouth and postural hypotension are present, and examination often shows an increase in strength (and augmentation of deep tendon reflexes) following exercise. Treatment with steroids and pyridostigmine can be helpful but events are usually overtaken by progression of the underlying malignancy.

Neurology

Muscle Disease

Ataxia

Q 19. Which of the following is not a recognised cause of ataxia?

  A. Carbamazepine toxicity
  B. Varicella zoster virus infection
  C. Small cell lung cancer
  D. Xeroderma pigmentosum
  E. Amyotrophic lateral sclerosis

Q 20. A 35-year-old man is diagnosed with multiple sclerosis. Which of the following statements would not be accurate advice about the likely course of his illness?

  A. Impotence is common
  B. The course is benign in 50%
  C. β-interferon is not indicated for primary progressive disease
  D. Steroid treatment hastens the resolution of an acute relapse
  E. The clinical state at diagnosis does not allow accurate prediction of the likely course of the illness

<u>A</u> **19. E**

<u>A</u> **20. B**

The majority of anti-epileptic drugs can cause ataxia if drug levels are excessive, especially phenytoin, and sometimes when levels are in the usual therapeutic range. Except with chronic phenytoin toxicity where a permanent cerebellar syndrome may occur, the symptoms resolve when levels fall into the normal range.

Varicella infection, usually in childhood, can cause an acute cerebellar syndrome.

Malignancies, especially small cell lung cancer, may be preceded or accompanied by a rapidly progressive cerebellar syndrome, sometimes associated with the presence of anti-neuronal or anti-Purkinje cell antibodies in the serum. CT often reveals cerebellar atrophy and there is a lymphocytic pleocytosis in the CSF. Treatment of the underlying malignancy does not alter the outcome of the disease although rarely immunosuppression or treatment with plasmapheresis may produce temporary improvement. Pathologically there is loss of Purkinje cells in the cerebellum.

Xeroderma pigmentosum is a rare disorder of DNA repair which is inherited in an autosomal recessive fashion. The commonest manifestation is severe photosensitivity with a predisposition to developing multiple cutaneous malignancies. Some patients develop a peripheral neuropathy and others may develop ataxia, dementia, deafness and movement disorders.

Ataxia
Most cases are caused by cerebellar dysfunction although it may also be produced by disorders of proprioception resulting from peripheral neuropathy or dorsal column disease. Frontal lobe lesions may produce a gait disorder, the so-called apraxic gait which can be difficult to distinguish from cerebellar ataxia. Midline cerebellar lesions produce eye movement abnormalities, gait ataxia and axial tremor, whereas peripheral lesions will produce dysmetria, dysdiadochokinesia, hypotonia in addition to the other abnormalities. Dysarthria does not localise well.

Causes
Congenital
- Cerebral palsy

Hereditary degenerative
- Friedrich's ataxia
- Early onset hereditary ataxias (usually AR)
- Late onset hereditary ataxias (usually AD)

Hereditary related to abnormalities in DNA repair
- Ataxia telangiectasia
- Cockayne syndrome
- Xeroderma pigmentosum

Hereditary metabolic
- Hyperammonaemias
- Aminoacidurias
- Abetalipoproteinaemia
- Storage disorders
- Leukodystrophies
- Wilson's disease
- Mitochondrial disease

Structural abnormalities
- Hydrocephalus
- Foramen magnum abnormalities

Tumours

Toxins
- Alcohol
- Heavy metals
- Organic solvents

Vitamin deficiencies
- Wernicke's encephalopathy
- Vitamin E deficiency

Drugs
- Anti-epileptics
- Lithium
- Cyclosporin A
- Cytotoxic agents

Demyelination
- Multiple sclerosis
- Acute disseminated encephalomyelitis

Paraneoplastic

Infarction/haemorrhage

Infection
- Measles
- Rubella
- HIV
- VZV
- Atypicals

Prion disease

Hypothyroidism

Multiple sclerosis is one of the commonest neurological diseases with an incidence of 130 per 100,000. The aetiology remains unknown although an environmental factor is implicated on epidemiological grounds. There is an association with the DR15/DQ6 haplotype. Pathologically, focal areas of demyelination in the brain are seen with evidence of macrophage and microglial activation and a predominantly Th1 cell-mediated inflammatory response. The precise relation of the inflammatory lesions to the axonal loss which is the main determinant of disability remains unresolved. Clinically, episodes of neurological dysfunction occurring in a relapsing-remitting fashion occur in 80%; 70% of those develop secondarily progressive disease at some point. Primary progressive disease occurs in 10% and the disease has a benign course in about 25%. The commonest sites of inflammatory plaques are optic nerve, brainstem, spinal cord, and cerebellum. Autonomic dysfunction occurs early. Investigations show oligoclonal bands in the CSF in 80%, mildly elevated protein, and occasionally a mild lymphocytic pleocytosis. Visual and auditory evoked potentials may be delayed. MRI shows periventricular high signal lesions on T2 weighted images, a low lesion load is associated with a better prognosis. Other good prognostic features are visual symptoms, young age at onset and long duration between first and second events. Acute relapses are commonly treated with steroids and although this may hasten recovery it does not alter the burden of disability. In patients with remitting-relapsing disease β-interferon treatment is associated with about a third fewer relapses and slower accrual of disability in the short to medium term. There is also evidence that it may reduce by a similar amount the risk of developing multiple sclerosis in patients with evidence of MS on imaging who are treated following their first episode of demyelination. The cost-benefit analysis remains controversial. Other treatments of more dubious benefit include glatiramer acetate and azathioprine.

Respiratory Medicine

Lung Tumours

Q 1.   A 40-year-old man is undergoing investigation for acromegaly.
MRI of the pituitary fossa is normal, but a routine chest
X-ray reveals a large centrally based mass. The patient is a
non-smoker. The most likely type of lung tumour is:

   A.   Squamous cell
   B.   Small cell
   C.   Carcinoid ✓
   D.   Large cell
   E.   Adenocarcinoma

Q 2.   A patient is diagnosed with primary adenocarcinoma of the left
upper lobe of the lung. The FEV$_1$ is 1.8 (60% predicted) and the
staging CT scan shows only ipsilateral hilar lymphadenopathy.
The next step for the patient is:

   A.   Chemotherapy
   B.   Radiotherapy and chemotherapy
   C.   Lobectomy
   D.   Mediastinoscopy and lobectomy ✓
   E.   Best supportive care

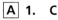

A 1. **C**

A central based mass in a non-smoker showing clinical evidence of neuroendocrine cell origin is consistent with a carcinoid. It represents the well differentiated spectrum of small cell lung cancer and surgery in non-metastatic disease confers 90% survival at 5 years.

A 2. **D**

The best chance of cure for someone with primary non-small cell lung cancer is surgery. CT is not always able to exclude mediastinal node involvement and mediastinoscopy is always required before surgery.

Para neoplastic syndromes in lung cancer
- Cerebellar syndrome – antineuronal antibodies are directed against the Purkinje cells of the cerebellum
- The Eaton-Lambert syndrome is a pre-synaptic disorder of autoantibody IgG directed against the pre-synaptic calcium channel leading to impaired acetylcholine release. Clinically patients present with muscle weakness that improves with exercise
- HPOA – most commonly with squamous cell cancer. HPOA does not occur with small cell lung cancer
- Hypercalcaemia – PTH-RP (squamous cell commonly)
- Hyponatraemia – SIADH (small cell commonly)

Surgery for non-small cell lung cancer (NSCLC)
NSCLC represents 80% of all lung cancers. 80% of these are clinically inoperable. Surgery confers a 40% survival at 5 years.

NSCLC is inoperable if:
- $FEV_1 < 1.5 l$ for lobectomy
- Mediastinal nodes or contra-lateral hilar nodes are enlarged (>1.5 cm)
- Pleural effusion or metastatic spread elsewhere is present
- Mediastinal structure involvement is present
- Satellite nodules are present in the same lobe or different lobe or lung

HIV and the Lung

Q 3. A 38-year-old HIV-positive man presents with life threatening haemoptysis. Which one of the following features would be consistent with Kaposi's sarcoma as the cause?

A. Pleural effusion ✓
B. Lack of systemic symptoms
C. Generalised lymphadenopathy
D. HIV acquired through IV drug abuse
E. Cavity on chest X-ray

Q 4. A patient with pneumocystis carinii pneumonia (PCP) has the following blood gases: PaO$_2$ 6.9 kPa and PaCO$_2$ 3.5 kPa. The most important prognostic step is:

A. Nasal ventilation
B. Physiotherapy
C. Intravenous steroids
D. Urgent commencement of retroviral therapy
E. Controlled oxygen therapy

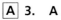

A 3. **A**

Kaposi's sarcoma (KS) is a very vascular tumour and a cause of life threatening haemoptysis. Pleural effusion is commonly involved with lung malignancy and in 30% of cases of KS. Systemic symptoms are common. The finding of generalised lymphadenopathy and cavitation is non-specific in HIV.

A 4. **C**

In pneumocystis carinii pneumonia, steroids decrease the risk of respiratory failure by 50%, and the risk of death by 33%. Steroids are indicated if the arterial oxygen tension is less than or equal to 9.3 kPa on air.

Common causes of respiratory disease in HIV are:
- *Pneumocystis carinii* (the most common opportunistic infection in HIV)
- *Mycobacterium tuberculosis*
- *Mycobacterium avium-intracellulare* (other atypical mycobacteria are rare)
- Organisms that commonly cause community acquired pneumonia – *Streptococcus pneumoniae, Haemophilus influenzae, Mycoplasma pneumoniae, Staphylococcus aureus.* In addition both Gram negative bacteria and *Brahmnella catarrhalis* are commonly seen
- Cytomegalovirus
- Other organisms including fungi and viruses are rare

Q 5. A 34-year-old woman presents with a prolonged history of epistaxis and rapidly progressive, shortness of breath. The KCO and eosinophil count are raised. The most likely diagnosis is:

    A. Goodpasture's syndrome
    B. Microscopic polyangiitis
    C. Churg-Strauss syndrome
    D. Wegener's granulomatosis ✓
    E. Alveolar proteinosis

Q 6. A 50-year-old patient with asthma is prescribed a leukotriene inhibitor. He presents with severe abdominal pain and a pleural effusion. The most likely cause of the effusion is:

    A. Carcinoma
    B. Pancreatitis
    C. Pneumonia
    D. Heart failure
    E. Churg-Strauss syndrome ✓

Respiratory Medicine

Systemic Disease and the Lung

A 5. D

A patient with breathlessness and a raised KCO has alveolar haemorrhage till proven otherwise. A prolonged history of epistaxis or sinusitis is commonly found in Wegener's granulomatosis, which in some patients is also associated with an eosinophilia. A history of asthma must usually be present to diagnose the Churg-Strauss syndrome.

A 6. E

Churg-Strauss syndrome has a predilection for serosal surfaces and therefore can cause both pleural and pericardial effusions and peritonitis. Cytological analysis of this fluid would confirm an eosinophilia. Leukotriene inhibitor use is associated with an increased incidence of the disease.

Name	Vasculitis of lung	ANCA finding
Large vessel vasculitis		
Giant cell (temporal) arteritis	Rare	None
Takayasu's arteritis	Frequent	None
Medium vessel vasculitis		
Polyarteritis nodosa	Rare	None
Kawasaki disease	None	None
Small vessel vasculitis		
Wegener's granulomatosis	Frequent	PR3-ANCA
Churg-Strauss syndrome	Frequent	MPO-ANCA or PR3-ANCA
Microscopic polyangiitis	Frequent	MPO-ANCA or PR3-ANCA
Henoch-Schönlein purpura	None	None
Essential cryoglobulinaemia	None	None

Community Acquired Pneumonia

Q 7. A 28-year-old builder is admitted with sudden onset high fever, left-sided pleuritic chest pain and confusion. This presentation is most suggestive of pneumonia caused by:

A. *Haemophilus influenzae*
B. *Mycoplasma pneumoniae*
C. *Streptococcus pneumoniae*
D. Influenza type A
E. *Legionella pneumophila*

Q 8. A 34-year-old plumber has just started treatment for a community acquired pneumonia but is noticed to have developed anaemia with a fall in haemoglobin of 3 g/dl over 7 days. The MCV is 102 fl. The most useful investigation is:

A. Mycoplasma serology
B. Reticulocyte count
C. Haematinic measurements
D. Liver function tests
E. Endoscopy

A 7. C

Streptococcus pneumoniae typically presents with acute onset, high fever and pleuritic chest pain. Elderly and patients with co-morbidity are at increased risk. Female sex, diabetes mellitus, COPD and alcoholism are associated with bacteraemia.

A 8. A

Anaemia with a macrocytosis in an acute setting suggests haemolysis. Although several of the options would help confirm this, the aetiology is best confirmed by mycoplasma serology. Haemolysis secondary to cold agglutins (IgM) is found with Mycoplasma pneumoniae infection and also infectious mononucleosis, large cell lymphoma and Waldenstrom's macroglobulinaemia.

Features of severe pneumonia
Clinical
- Respiratory rate ≥30 breaths/min
- Diastolic blood pressure <60 mmHg
- Confusion
- New-onset atrial fibrillation
- Multi-lobar involvement

Laboratory
- Serum albumin <35 g/l
- Serum urea >7 mmol/l
- PaO_2 <8 kPa on air or oxygen
- Bacteraemia
- Total white cell count <4 × 10^9/l or >20 × 10^9/l

Q 9. Which of the following additional features would be most suggestive of a diagnosis of cystic fibrosis in a young woman with recurrent chest infections?

A. A prolonged prothrombin time and high sweat sodium ✓
B. A high sweat sodium
C. Weight loss
D. Infertility
E. Haemoptysis

Q 10. A 24-year-old man is referred for investigation of the cause of chronic sputum production and haemoptysis. He is a non-smoker. The most appropriate next investigation is:

A. IgG subclass measurement
B. Electron microscopy (EM) of a nasal biopsy
C. Sweat test
D. Aspergillus IgG and IgE levels
E. High resolution computer tomography (HRCT) of the lungs

A 9. A

A prolonged prothrombin time would suggest both malabsorption of Vitamin K and cirrhosis, both specific complications of cystic fibrosis (CF). The other findings are also found in CF but are not specific to the disease.

A 10. E

Chronic production of sputum and haemoptysis is very consistent with underlying bronchiectasis. HRCT is diagnostic of the disease. Once the diagnosis is established the cause must be found.

Gastrointestinal complications of CF
- Meconium ileus equivalent (MIE) (treat with acetylcysteine and small bowel lavage)
- Increased incidence of GI malignancy
- Pancreatic insufficiency (malabsorption and diabetes mellitus, decreased stool trypsin activity)
- Cirrhosis (deranged liver function tests and prothrombin time)

Causes of bronchiectasis
Localised
- Severe pneumonia
- Foreign body obstruction of airway with recurrent infection as a result

Generalised
- Allergic bronchopulmonary aspergillosis (ABPA)
- Cystic fibrosis
- Ciliary dyskinetic syndromes (Young's and Kartagener's syndromes)
- Hypogammaglobulinaemia
- Defects of cartilage (Williams-Campbell and Mounier-Kuhn syndromes)
- Rheumatoid arthritis, SLE, Sjögren's syndrome
- Inflammatory bowel disease
- Yellow nail syndrome
- Marfan's and Ehlers-Danlos syndromes

Eosinophilia and the Lung

Q 11. An airline pilot presents with cough, wheeze and bloody sputum. The CXR shows upper lobe infiltrates and the eosinophil count is 1.2. The most important diagnostic step is:

    A. Sputum for acid-fast-bacilli
    B. Stool for ova, cysts and parasites
    C. Aspergillus IgE and IgG
    D. Bronchoscopy
    E. HIV testing

Q 12. A 24-year-old patient presents with cough, wheeze and low-grade fever. The eosinophil count is raised. Which of the following is the least likely diagnosis?

    A. Extrinsic allergic alveolitis
    B. Salicylate abuse
    C. Tropical pulmonary eosinophilia
    D. Churg-Strauss syndrome
    E. Allergic bronchopulmonary mycosis

A 11. C

ABPA is associated with eosinophilia, high aspergillus IgE (leads to positive skin prick tests), frequently positive aspergillus IgG (precipitins) and eosinophilic consolidation of the lung that is characteristically flitting in nature. Asthma and proximal bronchiectasis are clinical complications.

A 12. A

Extrinsic 'allergic' alveolitis is not associated with wheezing but with fever, coughing and dyspnoea. In addition, eosinophilia is not a feature. All the rest cause eosinophilia.

Causes of eosinophilia
- Infections
  - *Ascaris lumbricoides* (Loeffler's syndrome)
  - Microfilaria (tropical pulmonary eosinophilia)
  - *Toxocara canis* (visceral larva migrans)
  - Schistosoma species
- Atopy
- Drugs e.g. aspirin
- Allergic bronchopulmonary aspergillosis (ABPA)
- Churg – Strauss syndrome

Circulation of the Lung

Q 13. A 41-year-old man presents unwell. He is noted to have a
microcytic anaemia and pulse oximetry shows saturations of
89% on air. 48 h later he suffers a dense left hemiplegia.
There is a strong family history of stroke and several other
members of his immediate family have been anaemic. The
most likely diagnosis is:

    A. Hereditary haemorrhagic telangiectasia
    B. Vasculitis
    C. Pulmonary arterio-venous malformation
    D. Patent foramen ovale
    E. Ventricular septal defect

Q 14. A 37-year-old hairdresser who has been HIV-positive for 10 years
presents with progressive shortness of breath on exercise.
The chest X-ray is normal except for prominent pulmonary
arteries. Pulse oximetry shows he desaturates on exercise.
The most likely diagnosis is:

    A. *Pneumocystis carinii* pneumonia
    B. Primary pulmonary hypertension
    C. Intracardiac shunt across an atrial septal defect
    D. Pulmonary embolic disease
    E. Anaemia

A 13. A

Hypoxia and a history of stroke should suggest a right to left shunt. The history of anaemia and family history would be consistent with hereditary haemorrhagic telangiectasia (HHT) as they bleed from both cerebral and gut arterio-venous malformations.

A 14. B

Enlarged pulmonary central vasculature but otherwise normal chest X-ray suggests pulmonary arterial hypertension, a primary form of which is associated with chronic HIV infection. Pulmonary arterial hypertension should be suggested by enlargement of the central elastic arteries and pruning of the peripheral arteries. The pulmonary artery systemic pressure is usually >30 mmHg. Pulmonary oligaemia (the pulmonary trunk is small or inapparent with small peripheral vessels) usually indicates right ventricular outflow obstruction with a right to left shunt. Uneven vascularity on the CXR is expected with embolic disease.

Hereditary haemorrhagic telangiectasia
- Autosomal dominant
- Bleeding
  - Nose
  - Skin (telangiectasia)
  - Cerebral
  - GI
  - Lungs

Most of cerebral symptoms are due to pulmonary AVMs, with TIAS and abscesses due to presence of a R→L shunt.

Chronic Obstructive Airways Disease

Q 15. **A 52-year-old man with history of smoking presents with breathlessness. Spirometry shows an obstructive pattern. The most appropriate first line of treatment is:**

    A. Inhaled steroid
    B. High dose inhaled steroid to prevent disease progression
    C. Salbutamol
    D. Ipratropium bromide
    E. Salmeterol

Q 16. **Which of the following patterns of lung function tests would best fit someone with alpha-1 antitrypsin deficiency?**

    A. Obstructive spirometry with low KCO and MM genotype
    B. Obstructive spirometry, markedly decreased KCO and basal emphysema
    C. Obstructive spirometry, markedly decreased KCO and upper lobe emphysema
    D. Obstructive spirometry, normal KCO and basal emphysema
    E. Low KCO and normal residual volume

A 15. D

Anticholinergics are more effective than β₂ agonists in COPD and are thus the treatment of choice during the initiation of therapy. Steroids do not alter the progression of the disease (unlike asthma) and are reserved for patients who demonstrate steroid responsiveness or very severe disease.

A 16. B

Although COPD due to alpha-1 antitrypsin can present in any of the described ways the classic presentation is of predominantly basal emphysema and is pan-acinar (obstructive spirometry and low KCO). The PiZZ genotype leads to the worst form of the disease.

Reduced TLCO (transfer factor)
- Pneumonectomy
- Anaemia
- Interstitial lung disease
- COPD
- Vasculitis
- Extra thoracic restriction

Increased TLCO
- Alveolar haemorrhage
- Polycythaemia
- High output states (e.g. exercise)
- Acute asthma

Adult Respiratory Distress Syndrome

Q 17. The most important investigation to confirm the adult respiratory distress syndrome in an adult with refractory hypoxaemia is:

A. Chest X-ray
B. Echocardiogram
C. CT thorax
D. Pulmonary artery catheter with wedge pressure measurement ✓
E. Broncho-alveolar lavage

Q 18. In the adult respiratory distress syndrome the most important determinant of a good prognosis is:

A. Use of steroids
B. High PEEP settings to overcome decreased pulmonary compliance
C. Use of inotropes for cardiovascular support
D. The underlying cause of the syndrome ✓
E. Nutrition

A 17. D

The radiological investigations mimic heart failure in the adult respiratory distress syndrome (ARDS) and it is important to confirm that the pulmonary capillary wedge pressure (PCWP) is less than or equal to 18 mmHg (thus no evidence of left ventricular failure).

A 18. D

The management of ARDS is supportive and although this does effect prognosis, the overall survival rate is dependent on the cause.

Diagnostic criteria for ARDS
1. Acute onset
2. Widespread bilateral CXR infiltrates
3. Refractory hypoxaemia
4. PAWP <18 mmHg

Q 19. A patient with rheumatoid arthritis develops a progressive fall in the FEV_1. The residual volume is increased by 2l and the measurements of diffusion are normal. The patient is a smoker. The most likely diagnosis is:

A. Organising pneumonia
B. Bronchiolitis obliterans ✓
C. Caplan's syndrome
D. Rheumatoid associated lung fibrosis
E. Chronic obstructive pulmonary disease

Q 20. Which one of the following patients carries the highest risk of developing lymphoma of the lung?

A. A heavy smoker with recurrent chest infections
B. A woman with a 8 year history of dry eyes and mouth with nucleolar anti-nuclear antibody ✓
C. A patient with recurrent scarring alopecia
D. A man with seronegative spondyloarthropathy
E. A smoker with cough productive of copious quantities of sputum

A 19. **B**

Although all of the possible options can occur in rheumatoid arthritis, a progressive and relentless fall in the FEV_1 indicates bronchiolitis obliterans. Inflammation in the small distal airways leads to obstructive spirometry and this is relentlessly progressive. Air trapping occurs as a consequence leading to increased lung volumes.

A 20. **B**

Primary Sjögren's syndrome is associated with an increased incidence of lymphoid lung malignancy. Dry mouth and dry eyes is a classic symptom of this condition, and patients are ANA positive with a nucleolar pattern.

Physiology

Q 21. **A 45-year-old woman is breathless. The TLCO is very low but the KCO is 190% predicted. The most likely diagnosis is:**

A. Neuromuscular chest wall disorder
B. Primary pulmonary hypertension (PPH)
C. A patient with the ZZ genotype for alpha-1 antitrypsin
D. Scleroderma
E. Hereditary haemorrhagic telangiectasia

Q 22. **A 34-year-old man is rescued from a burning building and brought to hospital. He has nausea, vomiting, diarrhoea and abdominal pain. He is confused. The carboxy-haemoglobin (COHb) level is 25%. Which of the following is the best treatment for this patient?**

A. Hyperbaric oxygen
B. High flow oxygen via a facial mask
C. CT brain and lumbar puncture
D. Intravenous fluid and oxygen via nasal prongs
E. Urgent senior surgical opinion to exclude bowel obstruction

A 21. A

Patients with extra-pulmonary restriction (e.g. neuromuscular chest wall disorders) the lungs cannot fully inflate. Thus the surface area available for gaseous exchange is decreased (low TLCO). However, the cardiac output is unchanged so that a higher density of blood per unit volume is obtained resulting in a raised KCO.

A 22. A

Carboxy-haemoglobin (COHb) levels do not correlate well with the clinical picture. The indications for hyperbaric oxygen are neurological or psychiatric symptoms, cardiac complications, COHb levels of >40% and pregnant women.

CO binds with haemoglobin 230 times more tenacity than the oxygen so that a very marked leftward shift of the curve occurs.

Causes of rightward shift of the oxygen-haemoglobin dissociation curve
- Acidosis
- Hypercapnia
- Hyperthermia
- 2,3 DPG

Both severe illness and exercise create the above tissue conditions.

Asthma

Q 23. **The most important finding to confirm the diagnosis of asthma is:**

   A. High total blood IgE level
   B. Demonstration of airway reversibility
   C. High levels of interleukin-5 and granulocyte macrophage colony stimulating factor (GM-CSF) in blood
   D. Family history of asthma
   E. A high TLCO and KCO

Q 24. **A 20-year-old college student is referred with breathlessness. Exercise-induced asthma is the most likely diagnosis if:**

   A. Inhaled steroid abolishes the symptoms
   B. There is no history of atopy
   C. The symptoms usually occur at the end of strenuous exercise
   D. The symptoms re-occur on immediate repeat exercise
   E. Leukotriene receptor antagonist abolishes the symptoms

A 23. B

Asthma by definition must demonstrate variability in airflow limitation. The other investigations would suggest asthma but can also occur with other respiratory diseases.

A 24. E

Exercise-induced asthma is due to cold air drying the mucosa and affecting the periciliary fluid osmotics. This leads to inflammatory release and symptoms occur within 5–10 min of exercise and lasts up to 1 h. There is usually a refractory period following this of up to 2–4 h. Cysteinyl leukotrienes are key players here and leukotriene receptor antagonists are used to prevent exercise-induced bronchospasm. Steroids are not helpful.

Causes of occupational asthma
- Isocyanaces (paint, wire coating)
- Grain dust
- Colophony (from soldering flux)
- Epoxy resins (plastics, adhesives)
- Enzymes (detergents)
- Animals/insects (lab workers)

Granulomatous Lung Disease

Q 25. A 38-year-old man presents with severe arthralgia of the ankles and red swellings. The CXR shows bilateral hilar lymphadenopathy. The treatment of choice is:

A. Analgesia
B. High dose prednisolone ✓
C. High dose prednisolone and azathioprine
D. Observation
E. Inhaled steroid

Q 26. A 49-year-old miner develops smear positive *Mycobacterium tuberculosis*. Which of the following dusts is most likely to have increased the risk of this infection in this patient?

A. Coal dust
B. Asbestos
C. Cadmium
D. Silica ✓
E. Beryllium

A 25. B

Lofgren's syndrome. This is also known as Erythema Nodosum syndrome and is characterised by the abrupt onset of fever, arthralgia and erythema nodosum. There is bilateral hilar lymphadenopathy on the CXR and no other real lung involvement. This form of sarcoid is usually self-limiting and has an excellent prognosis with recurrence and any pulmonary involvement being rare. No steroid treatment is usually required, unless systemic symptoms are severe.

A 26. D

Silica is toxic to macrophages and impairs their function. Thus there is an increased risk of *Mycobacterium tuberculosis* in slate workers, stone masons, fettlers and miners (drilling through quartz strata).

Indications for immunosuppression in sarcoidosis
- Hypercalcaemia
- Ocular complications
- Cardiac complications
- Neurological complications
- Skin infiltration
- Progressive decrease in lung function
- Severe systemic symptoms

Therapeutics and the Lung

Q 27. **The most appropriate treatment regimen for a Russian man with smear positive mycobacterial disease is:**

   A. Isolation and rifampicin and ethambutol for 12 months
   B. BCG vaccination
   C. Rifampicin and isoniazid for 2 months and review sensitivity
   D. Rifampicin, pyrazinamide,ethambutol for 12 months
   E. Rifampicin, isoniazid, pyrazinamide, ethambutol for
       2 months and review sensitivity ✓

Q 28. **A 40-year-old window cleaner wants to quit smoking. He is on aspirin, a steroid inhaler and phenytoin. The best treatment for this man is:**

   A. Counselling
   B. Bupropion (Zyban™)
   C. Nicotine patches
   D. Counselling and nicotine patches ✓
   E. Fluoxetine

A 27. E

Multi-drug resistant (MDR)-TB is of concern in anyone who is from a part of the world where MDR-TB is prevalent and also in those who have had previous partially treated disease. Thus a 4 drug regime until sensitivity is available is usual practice.

A 28. D

Bupropion (Zyban™) is far more effective than nicotine patches in smoking cessation. However it is contra-indicated in patients with eating disorder and those with a history of seizures. There is no advantage in combining nicotine patches with bupropion.

Respiratory Failure

Q 29. A 58-year-old, obese, heavy smoker presents with impotence, nocturia and depression. He is hypoxic at rest on air and has ankle oedema. The most appropriate investigation to determine the aetiology is:

A. Arterial blood gas
B. Chest X-ray
C. Ventilation-perfusion scan
D. Thyroid function test
E. Sleep study ✓

Q 30. Long term oxygen therapy for an ex-smoker with Type II respiratory failure would best:

A. Improve lung function of the patient
B. Improve the quality of life of the patient
C. Prolong survival of the patient
D. Have no effect on the patient's haemoglobin level
E. Have the most benefit if used for episodes of shortness of breath only

A 29. E

Cor pulmonale secondary to diurnal respiratory failure occurs in patients with severe obstructive sleep apnoea (OSA). Most patients who develop this complication have lower airway obstruction (from smoking), gross obesity or respiratory muscle weakness. Hypercapnia out of proportion to the degree of lung disease should suggest OSA as a possible diagnosis.

A 30. C

Long term oxygen therapy (LTOT) in COPD leads to:

- Improved survival
- Improved polycythaemia
- Slowing of any further increases in pulmonary artery pressure
- No improvement in lung function occurs
- Quality of life remains unchanged

The benefit of LTOT is proportional to the number of hours per day the oxygen is worn by the patient.

Obstructive sleep apnoea associations
- Obesity
- Alcohol
- Acromegaly
- Hypothyroidism

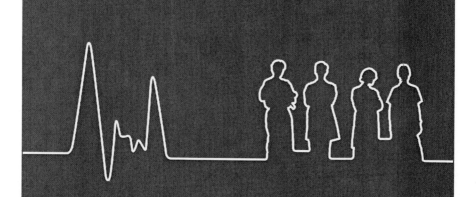

set your pulse racing

PULSE Doctors offer you nationwide placements, holiday pay and excellent rates for short or long term positions.

Let PULSE Doctors find the right position for you.

Keep up the pace and contact us today.

020 8989 1010 or email
enquiries@pulsedoctors.com

www.pulsedoctors.com

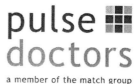

a member of the match group

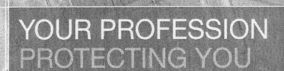